Quick and Easy
LOW GLYCEMIC
INDEX RECIPES

Quarto.com

© 2025 Quarto Publishing Group USA Inc.
Text © 2010 Dick Logue

First Published in 2025 by New Shoe Press, an imprint of The Quarto Group,
100 Cummings Center, Suite 265-D, Beverly, MA 01915, USA.
T (978) 282-9590 F (978) 283-2742

Essential, In-Demand Topics, Four-Color Design, Affordable Price
New Shoe Press publishes affordable, beautifully designed books covering evergreen, in-demand subjects. With a goal to inform and inspire readers' everyday hobbies, from cooking and gardening to wellness and health to art and crafts, New Shoe titles offer the ultimate library of purposeful, how-to guidance aimed at meeting the unique needs of each reader. Reimagined and redesigned from Quarto's best-selling backlist, New Shoe books provide practical knowledge and opportunities for all DIY enthusiasts to enrich and enjoy their lives.

Visit Quarto.com/New-Shoe-Press for a complete listing of the New Shoe Press books.

New Shoe Press titles are also available at discount for retail, wholesale, promotional, and bulk purchase. For details, contact the Special Sales Manager by email at specialsales@quarto.com or by mail at The Quarto Group, Attn: Special Sales Manager, 100 Cummings Center, Suite 265-D, Beverly, MA 01915, USA.

10 9 8 7 6 5 4 3 2 1

ISBN: 978-0-7603-9790-9
eISBN: 978-0-7603-9791-6

The content in this book was previously published in *500 Low-Glycemic Index Recipes* (Fair Winds Press) (2010) by Dick Logue.

Library of Congress Cataloging-in-Publication Data available

The information in this book is for educational purposes only. It is not intended to replace the advice of a physician or medical practitioner. Please see your health-care provider before beginning any new health program.

Printed in China

Quick and Easy
LOW GLYCEMIC INDEX RECIPES

Fight Diabetes and Heart Disease, Lose Weight, and Have Optimum Energy with Recipes That Let You Eat the Foods You Enjoy

DICK LOGUE

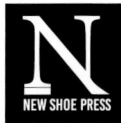

NEW SHOE PRESS

Contents

What Is a Low-Glycemic Index (GI) Diet?

Perhaps you've picked up this book because you've been hearing a lot lately about the glycemic index and how it can help you eat a more healthy diet. Perhaps you or someone you care about has diabetes, so things like carbohydrates, insulin production, and blood sugar levels are a special concern. Perhaps you are trying to lose weight and are confused about all the conflicting information about carbohydrates. Or perhaps you have one of my other books and are interested in what this new one had to offer. Maybe it's none of those reasons. Whatever the reason is, I can almost guarantee that there is information (and recipes!) here that will be useful to you.

I probably wouldn't have made that statement a year ago. I didn't know much about the glycemic index, other than that I thought it related to the amount of carbohydrates in food, and to be honest I wasn't very interested in it. I knew it was something that many doctors were talking about in relation to diabetic diets. But my mother had had diabetes for a number of years, and I thought from watching her and how she ate that I understood what was required to control your blood sugar level through diet. Basically she ate little or no sugar. She also was careful about not eating too many other carbohydrates, but not to an extreme. She still ate white bread with many meals as well as potatoes and other starches. This was common advice for people with diabetes when she was first diagnosed, and it worked pretty well for her. So I didn't give newer ideas much thought.

But my own doctor had been keeping a wary eye on my blood sugar levels, concerned that their slow rise from year to year and the family history of diabetes were signs that I would become diabetic myself. He suggested that I think about modifying my diet to be aware of the glycemic index values of the food I was eating as a way to help my body stabilize blood sugar levels. I wasn't really very happy with that suggestion. I already was on a low-sodium diet for congestive heart failure and about a year earlier had modified that diet to be aware of foods that could help me lower my cholesterol. It seemed like every time I had things pretty well worked out and was happy with what I could eat, it had to change because of some other factor.

But I dutifully began examining the facts about the glycemic index (often abbreviated GI) and how it related to the food we eat. I discovered that I hadn't really understood it, which didn't surprise me. However, I also discovered a lot of the foods that had been good things for fighting cholesterol were also low-GI foods. And I discovered that researchers were finding many benefits to low-GI foods beyond helping to stabilize blood sugar. And those things did surprise me. It was starting to sound like this might not be that difficult after all.

What Exactly Is the Glycemic Index?

The glycemic index does indeed relate to the carbohydrates in food. But it isn't so much a measure of the quantity of carbohydrates as their quality. Specifically it is a measure of how much the carbohydrates in foods affect your blood glucose level. Glucose is really what we are talking about when we use the term blood sugar as I did a few paragraphs ago. It is the most simple form of sugar, and its concentration in the blood is what we are measuring when we talk about "blood sugar levels." The digestive process converts other more complex sugars and starches, in other words carbohydrates, into glucose for use in the body. What the glycemic index measures is how quickly that process happens for different foods. High-GI foods break down quickly, causing a spike in the blood glucose level. Lower-GI foods break down more slowly but over a longer period of time, affecting blood glucose less.

The initial research on the glycemic index was done by Dr. David Jenkins and Dr. Thomas Wolever at the University of Toronto in the early 1980s. Prior to that time it was generally accepted that the diet my mother followed was the best for controlling blood sugar. It was believed that simple carbohydrates like granulated sugar broke down quickly and caused a sudden increase in blood glucose, while more complex carbohydrates like potatoes did not. Dr. Jenkins and his colleagues in Toronto tested a number of different foods, measuring the size and speed of their effect on blood glucose levels in the people eating them. He discovered that the common assumptions were not correct. In fact, some starches like potatoes, bread, and rice broke down much more quickly than the sugars in fruit and other foods.

The glycemic index for various foods was determined by testing people's blood glucose levels after they had eaten the foods. Pure glucose was assigned a value of 100, and other foods were given values based on how they raised the blood glucose level compared to glucose. Over the years a number of different studies have been done in Britain, France, Italy, Sweden, Australia, and Canada to determine the glycemic index of foods. Tables are available for over 700 different foods. While this isn't nearly every food, it does give us a good reference point for a lot of the more common foods containing carbohydrates. Foods such as meats, dairy products, and salad vegetables were not tested because they don't contain enough carbohydrates to raise the blood glucose level measurably. As expected, most foods have a GI value less than the 100 of pure glucose, although it was discovered that a few foods like jasmine rice actually affect the blood glucose level more than pure glucose. In general terms we call a food with a GI value of 55 or less low GI, 56 to 69 medium GI, and 70 or above high GI.

What Is the Difference between Glycemic Index and Glycemic Load?

You may also have heard the term glycemic load, or GL. This measure is related to, but different from, the glycemic index. The glycemic index is measured when a person eats a standard amount of a food, usually the amount containing 100 grams of carbohydrates, and the blood glucose response is measured. This gives us a good number to use in comparing foods.

However, some researchers realized that this can be misleading because a serving of a particular food does not usually contain exactly 100 grams of carbohydrates. Researchers at Harvard University came up with a new measure called glycemic load, which took this into consideration. The glycemic load is based on the glycemic index, adjusted for the normal serving size of the food.

An example of how this works might be an apple. An apple has a GI of 38, meaning that a serving of apples containing 100 grams of carbohydrates affects blood glucose 38 percent as much as 100 grams of glucose. But an apple only contains about 15 grams of carbohydrates. So eating one apple does not really affect blood glucose as much as the GI might indicate. The GL takes this into consideration by multiplying the GI of a food times the carbohydrates per serving, then dividing by 100. So the GL of an apple is 38 × 15 / 100 or about 6.

There is still some debate about whether GI or GL is a better measure of the quality of a food. On the one hand, GL takes the actual serving size into consideration, so it gives us a better picture of the actual affect on blood glucose of a particular food. However, people on the other side of the debate point out that the GL does not accurately tell you whether a food is one of the slow-acting ones that we are trying to eat more of. A food with a GI of 80 with a small serving size would have the same GL as a food with a GI of 40, but twice as large a portion. However, the food with the 80 GI would be the kind that is quickly digested, causing more of a spike in insulin levels and leaving us feeling hungry again sooner.

CHAPTER 1

What Should I Be Eating on a Low-GI Diet?

What Foods Are Low GI?

Let's get down to the real nitty-gritty of what foods you should be eating and what you should be avoiding in order to maintain a lower overall glycemic index. First let's look at some specific examples of the glycemic index of some foods, and then we'll talk about some general characteristics that tend to make a food lower or higher in GI. The values are taken from the studies done by Jennie Brand-Miller at the University of Sydney.

SOME LOW-GI FOODS (GI LESS THAN 55) AND THEIR GLYCEMIC INDEX

Yogurt, low fat (sweetened)	14	Grapefruit	25	Macaroni	45
Artichoke	15	Milk, whole	27	Rice, instant	46
Asparagus	15	Kidney beans, boiled	29	Grapes	46
Broccoli	15	Soy milk	30	Grapefruit juice	48
Cauliflower	15	Apricots (dried)	31	Multigrain bread	48
Celery	15	Milk, skim	32	Whole grain	50
Cucumber	15	Chickpeas	33	Barley, cracked	50
Eggplant	15	Spaghetti, whole wheat	37	Yam	51
Green beans	15	Apples	38	Orange juice	52
Lettuce, all varieties	15	Pears	38	Kiwifruit	53
Peppers, all varieties	15	Plums	39	Bananas	54
Snow peas	15	Carrots, cooked	39	Sweet potato	54
Spinach	15	Apple juice	41	Oat bran	55
Tomatoes	15	Wheat kernels	41	Rice, brown	55
Zucchini	15	Black-eyed beans	41	Fruit cocktail	55
Cherries	22	All-Bran	42	Spaghetti, durum wheat	55
Pearl barley	25	Peaches	42		
		Oranges	44		

SOME MEDIUM-GI FOODS (GI BETWEEN 56 AND 69) AND THEIR GLYCEMIC INDEX

Muesli	56	Rice, white	58	Pineapple	66
Mangoes	56	Danish pastry	59	Cake, angel	67
Potato, boiled	56	Pizza, cheese	60	Croissant	67
Pita bread, white	57	Hamburger bun	61	Taco shell	68
Rice, wild	57	Muffin (unsweetened)	62	Whole-meal bread	69
Apricots	57	Rye-flour bread	64	Shredded Wheat	69
Potato, new	57	Raisins	64	Potato, mashed	70
		Cake, tart	65		

SOME HIGH-GI FOODS (GI 70 AND ABOVE) AND THEIR GLYCEMIC INDEX

White bread	71	Waffles	76	Potato, baked	85
Golden Grahams	71	Doughnut	76	Baguette	95
Puffed Wheat	74	Rice Krispies	82	Parsnips	97
Potato chips	75	Cornflakes	83		

Looking down this list, we can begin to make some generalizations about the kinds of foods we should and should not be eating.

Changing to a Lower-GI Diet

So now that we've talked about the "why?" of a low-GI diet, the next obvious question is "how?". It's really not as difficult as you may be thinking. The short answer is that you need to become more aware of the GI range of the foods you are eating. I'm not going to tell you that you should never eat another high-GI item. I know that's not realistic.

What I am going to tell you is that you need to be careful about how often you eat high-GI foods and in what quantity. I'm going to give you recipes to help you think about low-GI foods that you can easily incorporate in to your diet and your family's. These are generally everyday things, the kind of food that you've been eating and liking all your life. But even if you use these recipes, you also need to think about the overall GI rating of everything you eat.

If you eat three or four low- to medium-GI foods in a meal, the total amount of carbohydrates and the GI rating for the entire meal will be pretty high. So you need to balance those things that have a moderate amount of carbohydrates and GI rating with some things that are at the low end of the scale.

One of the questions many people may have is the relationship of a low-GI diet to the popular low-carb diets. Plans like the Atkins diet have been popular in recent years, and some people have experienced success losing weight on them. However, there is also a high incidence of gaining weight back once you begin to ease up on the dietary restrictions. And a number of medical authorities question whether severe restriction of carbohydrates and the amount of fat many people eat to help replace the carbs is healthy over a long period of time.

What we are looking for here is a diet for the rest of your life. A diet that leaves you feeling satisfied with both the quantity, and perhaps even more importantly, the taste of the foods you eat. I can tell you from personal experience that one of the things that has pleased me the most about eating a lower-GI diet was finding that the flavor of things like whole grain breads and pasta and brown rice was actually better than the bland taste of their more refined, less healthy alternatives. The changes we are talking about are not going to make you aware of the restrictions; they are going to make you aware of how good healthy food can be.

Putting It All Together

I'm suggesting we set target daily goals of five to seven servings of vegetables, three to five servings of fruit, and limit the high-carb foods to three to eight servings. The next thing I'm going to suggest is that we try to eat foods that have gone through the least possible amount of processing. Here are a few examples:

- Choose whole grains over refined grains. Multigrain bread has a GI of 48, compared to 71 for white bread. Whole wheat spaghetti has a GI of 37, while regular durum wheat spaghetti has 55. And as I said, you'll find that whole grain products also have more flavor. It's a win-win situation.

- Choose raw fruits and vegetables over processed ones as much as possible. Raw fruit generally has more nutrients and a longer digestive cycle than canned fruit. Canned fruit has the same advantage over fruit juice. Raw vegetables are similarly better than cooked or canned ones. When you cook vegetables, steam or stir-fry them quickly until just crisp-tender to retain as much of the nutrition as possible.

Even though we're focusing here on carbohydrates and GI, be aware of other nutritional considerations. Meat does not contain enough carbohydrates to be an issue, but depending on the kind of meat and the cut it can contain a lot of saturated fat. Not only is that bad from a heart health and cholesterol standpoint, but if you're trying to maintain a healthy weight (and aren't we all), fat contains nearly twice the number of calories per gram as protein or carbs. Let's not get so focused on carbs that we don't remember the other things that make a diet healthy. In general, what many experts now think is the healthiest diet is one that is high in fiber and high in carbohydrates, but low in GI and low in fat. The bottom line in doing this is that just as all fats are not created equal and we have learned to cut down on saturated fats and trans fats, so all carbohydrates are not equal. We need to concentrate on choosing wisely. What we are looking for is not no carbs, but the right quantity of the right kind of carbs—those that are low on the glycemic index scale.

CHAPTER 2

Sauces and Condiments

Sauces and condiments are not generally a big concern from a GI standpoint. Most contain few carbohydrates. But there are other concerns, like the amount of sodium that many contain. What I've included here are some ideas that may help you think healthy and are very low in GI. They include reduced-sodium soy and teriyaki sauces, some other sauces that you won't find on your grocer's shelves, and some condiments to go with your new healthy meals.

Reduced-Sodium Soy Sauce

6 CALORIES (13% FROM FAT, 11% FROM PROTEIN, 76% FROM CARB)

Even though sodium is not a problem from a glycemic index standpoint, it is definitely connected to heart health and other medical problems. Soy sauce, even the reduced-sodium kinds, contains more sodium than many people's diet can stand. A teaspoonful often contains at least a quarter of the amount of sodium that is recommended for a healthy adult. If you have heart disease or are African American, the recommendation is even less. This sauce gives you real soy sauce flavor while holding the sodium to a level that should fit in most people's diet.

4 tablespoons (24 g) sodium-free beef bouillon

4 tablespoons (60 ml) cider vinegar

2 tablespoons (40 g) molasses

1½ cups (355 ml) water, boiling

⅛ teaspoon black pepper

⅛ teaspoon ginger

¼ teaspoon garlic powder

¼ cup (60 ml) reduced-sodium soy sauce

—

Yield: 48 servings

Combine ingredients, stirring to blend thoroughly. Pour into jars. Cover and seal tightly. This may be kept refrigerated indefinitely.

NUTRITIONAL ANALYSIS

EACH WITH: 10 g water; 0 g protein; 0 g total fat; 0 g saturated fat; 0 g monounsaturated fat; 0 g polyunsaturated fat; 1 g carb; 0 g fiber; 1 g sugar; 3 mg phosphorus; 4 mg calcium; 0 mg iron; 52 mg sodium; 19 mg potassium; 3 IU vitamin A; 0 mg vitamin C; 0 mg cholesterol

Reduced-Sodium Teriyaki Sauce

37 CALORIES (2% FROM FAT, 0% FROM PROTEIN, 98% FROM CARB)

The story on this recipe is the same as the soy sauce. In this case, you can sometimes find some commercial teriyaki sauces that aren't too high in sodium. But this one is much lower and to my mind tastes as good if not better.

1 cup (235 ml) Reduced-Sodium Soy Sauce (see recipe on facing page)

1 tablespoon (15 ml) sesame oil

2 tablespoons (30 ml) mirin wine

½ cup (100 g) sugar

3 cloves garlic, crushed

2 slices gingerroot

Dash black pepper

—

Yield: 20 servings

Combine all ingredients in a saucepan and heat until sugar is dissolved. Store in the refrigerator.

NUTRITIONAL ANALYSIS

EACH WITH: 17 g water; 0 g protein; 1 g total fat; 0 g saturated fat; 0 g monounsaturated fat; 2 g polyunsaturated fat; 84 g carb; 0 g fiber; 7 g sugar; 10 mg phosphorus; 7 mg calcium; 0 mg iron; 83 mg sodium; 32 mg potassium; 5 IU vitamin A; 0 mg vitamin C; 0 mg cholesterol

TIP

You can substitute sherry or saki for the mirin, a sweet Japanese rice wine.

Chili Sauce

12 CALORIES (1% FROM FAT, 1% FROM PROTEIN, 98% FROM CARB)

I've got to admit I've never been a really big fan of bottled chili sauce. The kids used it on hot dogs for a while, but I've always been a mustard and relish type of guy. Anyway, I much prefer the flavor of this chili sauce, which was adapted from a recipe from the American Heart Association to the kind found in stores. There are enough veggies in it to give it something more than a glorified ketchup taste. It keeps well in the refrigerator for weeks and you could freeze it if you wanted. The serving size for the nutritional calculation is 1 tablespoon.

1 can (14½ ounces or 410 g) no-salt-added tomatoes

1 can (8 ounces or 225 g) no-salt-added tomato sauce

½ cup (80 g) chopped onion

½ cup (100 g) sugar

½ cup (50 g) chopped celery

½ cup (75 g) chopped green pepper

1 tablespoon (15 ml) lemon juice

1 tablespoon (15 g) brown sugar

1 tablespoon (20 g) molasses

¼ teaspoon hot pepper sauce

⅛ teaspoon cloves

⅛ teaspoon cinnamon

⅛ teaspoon black pepper

⅛ teaspoon basil

⅛ teaspoon tarragon

½ cup (120 ml) cider vinegar

—
Yield: 48 servings

Combine all ingredients in a large saucepan. Bring to boil, reduce heat, and simmer uncovered 1½ hours or until mixture is reduced to half the original volume.

NUTRITIONAL ANALYSIS

EACH WITH: 0 g protein; 0 g total fat; 0 g saturated fat; 0 g monounsaturated fat; 3 g carb; 0 g fiber; 2 mg calcium; 0 mg iron; 2 mg sodium; 19 mg potassium; 12 IU vitamin A; 2 mg vitamin C; 0 mg cholesterol

Tomato Chutney

63 CALORIES (3% FROM FAT, 6% FROM PROTEIN, 91% FROM CARB)

This makes a great-tasting chutney. It's pretty spicy, so you may want to adjust the number of jalapeños.

1 cup (235 ml) cider vinegar

½ cup (12 g) sugar substitute, such as Splenda

1½ pounds (680 g) cherry tomatoes, quartered

2 cups (320 g) chopped onion

4 jalapeño peppers, chopped

2 teaspoons (4 g) ginger

2 cloves garlic, minced

1 teaspoon cumin

½ teaspoon cinnamon

½ cup (75 g) golden raisins

—

Yield: 16 servings

Combine vinegar and sugar in nonaluminum saucepan. Bring to a boil, stirring to dissolve sugar. Add remaining ingredients. Bring to a boil, reduce heat, and simmer 30 to 45 minutes, or until most of the liquid has cooked off. Stir often to prevent sticking. Refrigerate for up to 2 weeks or separate into containers and freeze.

NUTRITIONAL ANALYSIS

EACH WITH: 37 g water; 1 g protein; 0 g total fat; 0 g saturated fat; 0 g monounsaturated fat; 0 g polyunsaturated fat; 15 g carb; 1 g fiber; 10 g sugar; 23 mg phosphorus; 17 mg calcium; 1 mg iron; 3 mg sodium; 230 mg potassium; 272 IU vitamin A; 11 mg vitamin C; 0 mg cholesterol

CHAPTER 3

Appetizers, Snacks, and Party Foods

When many people think of snacks, the first thing they think of is chips and crackers, which are not good GI choices. Instead, use the recipes in this chapter to think about veggies, bean dips, and high-protein snacks. Many of these are fancy enough and tasty enough to serve at any party. But why wait? They are also easy enough to make for everyday use.

Teriyaki Chicken Nibbles

193 CALORIES (11% FROM FAT, 45% FROM PROTEIN, 43% FROM CARB)

These tasty little chicken fingers are always a hit as an appetizer or buffet item. The Asian flavor is a surprise, since they don't look any different from ordinary chicken fingers.

½ cup (120 ml) water

¾ cup (175 g) Reduced-Sodium Soy Sauce (see chapter 2)

¼ teaspoon garlic powder

1 teaspoon sugar

½ teaspoon ginger

1 pound (455 g) boneless skinless chicken breast

1½ cups (175 g) bread crumbs

—

Yield: 6 servings

Combine water, soy sauce, garlic powder, and ginger. Cut chicken into pieces approximately 2 × 1 × ½ inch (5 × 2½ × 1¼ cm). Marinate in soy sauce mixture for 2 hours. Drain. Coat pieces with bread crumbs. Deep fat fry in vegetable oil at 375°F (190°C) for about 1 minute. Drain on absorbent towels.

NUTRITIONAL ANALYSIS

EACH WITH: 78 g water; 21 g Protein; 2 g total fat; 1 g saturated fat; 1 g monounsaturated fat; 1 g polyunsaturated fat; 20 g carb; 1 g fiber; 2 g sugar; 193 mg phosphorous; 59 mg calcium; 2 mg iron; 50 mg sodium; 249 mg potassium; 16 IU vitamin A; 5 mg ATE vitamin E; 1 mg vitamin C; 44 mg cholesterol

Scotch Eggs

300 CALORIES (71% FROM FAT, 23% FROM PROTEIN, 6% FROM CARB)

These are a classic finger food. They can be served whole, halved, or quartered.

1½ pounds (675 g) sausage

12 eggs, hard cooked
and peeled

1 egg, beaten

½ cup (60 g) dry bread crumbs

—

Yield: 12 servings

Preheat oven to 450°F (230°C, or gas mark 8). Divide sausage into 12 equal portions; shape into patties. Wrap each sausage patty completely around 1 hard cooked egg, pressing edges together to seal. Dip sausage wrapped eggs in beaten egg; roll in bread crumbs until completely coated. Place in ungreased 15 × 10-inch (38 × 25 cm) jelly roll pan. Bake at 450°F (230°C, or gas mark 8) for 30 minutes or until meat is thoroughly browned and cooked.

NUTRITIONAL ANALYSIS

EACH WITH: 73 g water; 17 g Protein; 24 g total fat; 8 g saturated fat; 11 g monounsaturated fat; 3 g polyunsaturated fat; 4 g carb; 0 g fiber; 1 g sugar; 212 mg phosphorous; 49 mg calcium; 2 mg iron; 560 mg sodium; 224 mg potassium; 301 IU vitamin A; 85 mg ATE vitamin E; 0 mg vitamin C; 298 mg cholesterol

Chicken Wontons

48 CALORIES (23% FROM FAT, 26% FROM PROTEIN, 51% FROM CARB)

These tasty little chicken snacks are actually easier to make than they sound, and they are always a big hit.

8 ounces (225 g) ground chicken

½ cup (55 g) carrots, shredded

¼ cup (25 g) celery, finely chopped

1 tablespoon (15 g) Reduced-Sodium Soy Sauce (see chapter 2)

1 tablespoon (15 ml) sherry

2 teaspoons (5 g) cornstarch

2 teaspoons (4 g) ginger root

8 ounces (225 g) wonton wrappers

2 tablespoons (28 g) unsalted butter, melted

—

Yield: 25 servings

In a medium skillet cook and stir ground chicken until no pink remains; drain. Stir in carrots, celery, soy sauce, sherry, cornstarch, and ginger root; mix well. Spoon 1 rounded teaspoon of the filling atop a wonton wrapper. Lightly brush edges with water. To shape each wonton, carefully bring 2 opposite points of the square wrapper up over the filling and pinch together in the center. Carefully bring the 2 remaining opposite points to the center and pinch together. Pinch together edges to seal. Place wontons on a greased baking sheet. Brush the wontons with melted butter. Bake in a 375°F (190°C, or gas mark 5) oven for 8 to 10 minutes or until lightly brown and crisp.

NUTRITIONAL ANALYSIS

EACH WITH: 13 g water; 3 g Protein; 1 g total fat; 1 g saturated fat; 0 g monounsaturated fat; 0 g polyunsaturated fat; 6 g carb; 0 g fiber; 0 g sugar; 27 mg phosphorous; 7 mg calcium; 0 mg iron; 61 mg sodium; 43 mg potassium; 466 IU vitamin A; 9 mg ATE vitamin E; 0 mg vitamin C; 9 mg cholesterol

TIP

Serve these with salsa and fat-free sour cream.

Stuffed Mushrooms

43 CALORIES (33% FROM FAT, 48% FROM PROTEIN, 19% FROM CARB)

This makes a very nice appetizer for entertaining. It's fancy looking and tasting but still healthy.

¼ cup (25 g) minced scallions

2 teaspoons unsalted butter

1 can (4 ounces or 115 g) crabmeat, drained

2 tablespoons (8 g) minced fresh parsley

1 tablespoon (15 g) horseradish

2 cloves garlic, pressed

¼ teaspoon hot pepper sauce

2½ cups (145 g) mushroom caps (24), stems removed

Ground red pepper for garnish

—
Yield: 6 servings

Combine scallions and butter in 2-cup measure. Microwave on high 2 minutes; stir in crabmeat, parsley, horseradish, garlic, and pepper sauce. Stir well. Place half the mushrooms, stemmed sides up, in a 9-inch (23 cm) pie plate. Fill each mushroom cap with 1 teaspoon crab mixture. Microwave on high 3 to 4 minutes, turning plate once. Remove mushrooms to serving plate; repeat with remaining mushrooms and filling. Let stand 2 to 3 minutes before serving. To garnish, sprinkle with ground red pepper. Each serving contains 4 mushrooms.

NUTRITIONAL ANALYSIS

EACH WITH: 49 g water; 5 g protein; 2 g total fat; 1 g saturated fat; 0 g monounsaturated fat; 0 g polyunsaturated fat; 2 g carb; 1 g fiber; 1 g sugar; 20 mg calcium; 0 mg iron; 83 mg sodium; 198 mg potassium; 209 IU vitamin A; 5 mg vitamin C; 18 mg cholesterol

Green Onion Dip

17 CALORIES (5% FROM FAT,
79% FROM PROTEIN, 17% FROM CARB)

This is not at all like the packaged onion dip mixes, but it's still very tasty. It has a little more tang and is great to dip veggies in.

1 cup (225 g) cottage cheese

¼ cup (25 g) chopped green onion

2 teaspoons (10 ml) lemon juice

—

Yield: 8 servings

Combine ingredients in a blender or food processor and process until smooth. Refrigerate for at least an hour to give the flavors time to develop.

NUTRITIONAL ANALYSIS

EACH WITH: 18 g water; 3 g protein; 0 g total fat; 0 g saturated fat; 0 g monounsaturated fat; 0 g polyunsaturated fat; 1 g carb; 0 g fiber; 0 g sugar; 20 mg phosphorus; 8 mg calcium; 0 mg iron; 3 mg sodium; 16 mg potassium; 37 IU vitamin A; 1 mg vitamin C; 1 mg cholesterol

Hummus

155 CALORIES (41% FROM FAT,
15% FROM PROTEIN, 44% FROM CARB)

Hummus is a traditional Middle Eastern dip. I usually cook my own dried chickpeas, which you should be able to find with the other dried beans in most large markets. They are lower in sodium than the canned ones.

1 cup (164 g) cooked chickpeas

3 cloves garlic

3 tablespoons (45 ml) lemon juice

¼ cup (60 ml) water

¼ cup (60 g) tahini

1 teaspoon cumin

½ teaspoon paprika

1 tablespoon (15 ml) olive oil

—

Yield: 8 servings

Place the cooked chickpeas in the food processor along with the garlic, lemon juice, and water. Process for about a minute until smooth. If it's too thick, add more water. Stir in the tahini and spices, taste, and add more lemon juice/tahini/cumin/paprika as desired. Spread into a shallow bowl; drizzle with olive oil. Serve chilled.

NUTRITIONAL ANALYSIS

EACH WITH: 16 g water; 6 g protein; 7 g total fat; 1 g saturated fat; 3 g monounsaturated fat; 3 g polyunsaturated fat; 18 g carb; 5 g fiber; 3 g sugar; 63 mg calcium; 2 mg iron; 16 mg sodium; 269 mg potassium; 102 IU vitamin A; 4 mg vitamin C; 0 mg cholesterol

Bean Dip

151 CALORIES (26% FROM FAT, 23% FROM PROTEIN, 52% FROM CARB)

This makes a great bean and cheese dip that not only tastes better than commercial ones but is healthier besides.

2 tablespoons (30 ml) olive oil

½ teaspoon crushed garlic

1 cup (160 g) finely chopped onion

1 jalapeño pepper, finely chopped

1 teaspoon chili powder

2 cups (200 g) cooked kidney beans

½ cup (58 g) shredded cheddar cheese

—
Yield: 12 servings

Heat oil in a skillet. Add garlic, onion, jalapeño, and chili powder and cook gently 4 minutes. Drain kidney beans, reserving juice. Process beans in a blender or food processor to a puree. Add to onion mixture and stir in 2 tablespoons (30 ml) of reserved bean liquid; mix well. Stir in cheese. Cook gently about 2 minutes, stirring until cheese melts. If mixture becomes too thick, add a little more reserved bean liquid. Spoon into serving dish and serve warm with tortilla chips.

NUTRITIONAL ANALYSIS

EACH WITH: 19 g water; 9 g protein; 4 g total fat; 2 g saturated fat; 1 g monounsaturated fat; 1 g polyunsaturated fat; 20 g carb; 8 g fiber; 1 g sugar; 158 mg phosphorus; 87 mg calcium; 3 mg iron; 44 mg sodium; 463 mg potassium; 126 IU vitamin A; 3 mg vitamin c; 6 mg cholesterol

Guacamole Dip

80 CALORIES (46% FROM FAT, 30% FROM PROTEIN, 24% FROM CARB)

This recipe makes a lighter version of guacamole. It is a molded dip made with lemon gelatin.

1 small lemon flavor sugar-free gelatin

1 cup (235 ml) boiling water

¼ cup (60 ml) lemon juice

16 ounces (455 g) fat free cottage cheese

2 cloves garlic

2 teaspoons (5.2 g) chili powder

1 cup (146 g) avocado

¼ cup (45 g) tomatoes, finely chopped

½ cup (50 g) green onion, chopped, divided

4 pitted ripe olives, sliced

¼ cup (34 g) pickled jalapeno pepper

—
Yield: 10 servings

Completely dissolve gelatin in boiling water; pour into blender container. Add cottage cheese, avocado, half of the green onions, the jalapeno peppers, lemon juice, garlic, and chili powder. Cover and blend on low speed, scraping down sides occasionally, about 2 minutes or until mixture is smooth. Pour into shallow 5-cup (1.2 L) serving dish; smooth top. Chill until set, about 4 hours. When ready to serve, top guacamole with the remaining ¼ cup (25 g) chopped green onion, the tomatoes, and olives. Serve as a dip with chips or vegetables.

NUTRITIONAL ANALYSIS

EACH WITH: 93 g water; 6 g Protein; 4 g total fat; 1 g saturated fat; 3 g monounsaturated fat; 0 g polyunsaturated fat; 5 g carb; 2 g fiber; 2 g sugar; 86 mg phosphorous; 39 mg calcium; 0 mg iron; 214 mg sodium; 196 mg potassium; 290 IU vitamin A; 5 mg ATE vitamin E; 7 mg vitamin C; 2 mg cholesterol

Tofu Avocado Dip

54 CALORIES (63% FROM FAT, 15% FROM PROTEIN, 22% FROM CARB)

When you have an avocado and you are tired of guacamole, try this flavorful dip. The taste is vaguely Middle Eastern or Asian, but it really isn't quite like any other dip I've ever had. It can also be used as is for a tasty vegetarian sandwich filling.

8 ounces (225 g) tofu

½ cup (23 g) avocado

2 garlic cloves, chopped

2 teaspoons (4 g) minced fresh ginger

½ cup (30 g) fresh parsley leaves

2 tablespoons (30 ml) lemon juice

1 tablespoon (16 g) peanut butter

1 tablespoon (15 g) applesauce

—
Yield: 8 servings

Blend all ingredients in a food processor until very smooth.

NUTRITIONAL ANALYSIS

EACH WITH: 41 g water; 2 g protein; 4 g total fat; 1 g saturated fat; 2 g monounsaturated fat; 1 g polyunsaturated fat; 3 g carb; 1 g fiber; 1 g sugar; 32 mg phosphorous; 12 mg calcium; 0 mg iron; 3 mg sodium; 145 mg potassium; 22 IU vitamin A; 0 mg ATE vitamin E; 3 mg vitamin C; 0 mg cholesterol

Chili Horseradish Dip

27 CALORIES (4% FROM FAT, 36% FROM PROTEIN, 60% FROM CARB)

This is a flavorful dip for vegetables. We also like it as a salad dressing.

1 cup (230 g) plain fat-free yogurt

2 tablespoons (30 ml) chili sauce, see recipe in chapter 2

2 tablespoons (10 g) horseradish

—

Yield: 6 servings

Mix all ingredients; cover and refrigerate at least 1 hour.

NUTRITIONAL ANALYSIS

EACH WITH: 44 g water; 2 g Protein; 0 g total fat; 0 g saturated fat; 0 g monounsaturated fat; 0 g polyunsaturated fat; 4 g carb; 0 g fiber; 4 g sugar; 66 mg phosphorous; 85 mg calcium; 0 mg iron; 81 mg sodium; 116 mg potassium; 87 IU vitamin A; 1 mg ATE vitamin E; 3 mg vitamin C; 1 mg cholesterol

Crab Dip

245 CALORIES (74% FROM FAT, 23% FROM PROTEIN, 3% FROM CARB)

This crab dip has become a standard part of our Thanksgiving meal, giving people something to nibble on while dinner is being finished.

1 cup (230 g) sour cream

8 ounces (225 g) cream cheese

1 pound (455 g) crab meat

1 teaspoon dry mustard

¼ teaspoon garlic powder

¼ cup (60 g) mayonnaise

1 teaspoon old bay seasoning

1 cup (120 g) grated cheddar cheese

—

Yield: 10 servings

Cream all ingredients except crab meat and half of the cheese. Add crab meat and stir gently to combine. Sprinkle reserved cheese on top. Bake at 325°F (170°C, or gas mark 3) for 20 minutes.

NUTRITIONAL ANALYSIS

EACH WITH: 73 g water; 14 g Protein; 20 g total fat; 10 g saturated fat; 5 g monounsaturated fat; 3 g polyunsaturated fat; 2 g carb; 0 g fiber; 0 g sugar; 220 mg phosphorous; 180 mg calcium; 1 mg iron; 323 mg sodium; 224 mg potassium; 546 IU vitamin A; 145 mg ATE vitamin E; 2 mg vitamin C; 86 mg cholesterol

Dried Beef Appetizer Dip

107 CALORIES (78% FROM FAT, 16% FROM PROTEIN, 6% FROM CARB)

I don't use dried chipped beef very often because of the high sodium content. But for your guests who aren't watching their sodium, this is an excellent choice with a lot of flavor.

8 ounces (225 g) cream cheese, softened

2 tablespoons (30 ml) milk

2½ ounces (70 g) sliced dried beef, finely snipped

2 tablespoons (20 g) minced onion

2 tablespoons (19 g) green pepper, finely chopped

⅛ teaspoon pepper

½ cup (115 g) sour cream

¼ cup (30 g) walnuts, coarsely chopped

—
Yield: 12 servings

Blend cream cheese and milk. Stir in dried beef, onion, green pepper, and pepper; mix well. Stir in sour cream. Spoon into 8-inch (20 cm) pie plate or small shallow baking dish. Sprinkle walnuts over top. Bake at 350°F (180°C, or gas mark 4) for 15 minutes. Serve hot with assorted crackers.

NUTRITIONAL ANALYSIS

EACH WITH: 27 g water; 4 g Protein; 9 g total fat; 5 g saturated fat; 3 g monounsaturated fat; 1 g polyunsaturated fat; 2 g carb; 0 g fiber; 0 g sugar; 58 mg phosphorous; 31 mg calcium; 0 mg iron; 226 mg sodium; 76 mg potassium; 305 IU vitamin A; 79 mg ATE vitamin E; 2 mg vitamin C; 29 mg cholesterol

Papaya-Pineapple Salsa

23 CALORIES (2% FROM FAT, 5% FROM PROTEIN, 93% FROM CARB)

This fruity salsa is only mildly spicy, but it has great flavor. We like it best over fish, but try it with chicken or over a salad too.

¾ cup (135 g) ripe papaya, diced

¾ cup (120 g) fresh pineapple, diced

½ cup (65 g) jicama, diced

3 tablespoons (30 g) red onion

1 chili pepper, seeded and minced

1 clove garlic, minced

2 teaspoons (4 g) lime peel

2 tablespoons (30 ml) fresh lime juice

1 tablespoon (1 g) cilantro, minced

—
Yield: 8 servings

Combine papaya, pineapple, jicama, red onion, chili pepper, garlic, lime zest, lime juice, and cilantro. Cover and refrigerate until ready to serve. For best flavor and texture, do not make more than 2 hours before serving.

NUTRITIONAL ANALYSIS

EACH WITH: 46 g water; 0 g Protein; 0 g total fat; 0 g saturated fat; 0 g monounsaturated fat; 0 g polyunsaturated fat; 6 g carb; 1 g fiber; 4 g sugar; 6 mg phosphorous; 9 mg calcium; 0 mg iron; 1 mg sodium; 83 mg potassium; 196 IU vitamin A; 0 mg ATE vitamin E; 13 mg vitamin C; 0 mg cholesterol

CHAPTER 4

Breakfast

Breakfast can be a carbohydrate nightmare, with pancakes, waffles, and white bread toast. This chapter includes some lower-GI ideas. There are breakfast skillet and casserole dishes that feature mostly eggs, meat, and vegetables. There are grab-and-go ideas wrapped in tortillas rather than bread. And there are high-protein, low-carb smoothies that will keep you satisfied throughout the morning.

Sun-Dried Tomato Scrambled Eggs

148 CALORIES (61% FROM FAT, 27% FROM PROTEIN, 12% FROM CARB)

Sun-dried tomatoes turn ordinary scrambled eggs into a different taste treat. This recipe is perfect for those mornings when you want something a little different, but you don't know what.

4 eggs

¼ cup (60 ml) skim milk

½ teaspoon dried parsley

¼ cup (30 g) cheddar cheese, shredded

½ cup (27 g) sun-dried tomatoes

—

Yield: 4 servings

If using dried tomatoes, boil water in pot. Turn off heat and place tomatoes in water for about 3 minutes until soft. Cut up tomatoes in small pieces. Beat together eggs and milk. Place egg mixture in greased skillet. Add tomato pieces, cheese, and parsley. Scramble until done.

NUTRITIONAL ANALYSIS

EACH WITH: 67 g water; 10 g Protein; 10 g total fat; 4 g saturated fat; 4 g monounsaturated fat; 1 g polyunsaturated fat; 5 g carb; 1 g fiber; 1 g sugar; 184 mg phosphorous; 115 mg calcium; 1 mg iron; 173 mg sodium; 323 mg potassium; 577 IU vitamin A; 108 mg ATE vitamin E; 14 mg vitamin C; 246 mg cholesterol

Breakfast Wraps

Use this recipe on those days when you want a little something different for breakfast. This is similar to the breakfast burritos served at several fast food restaurants but with a lot less fat.

½ pound (225 g) turkey sausage

½ cup (80 g) onion, chopped

1 teaspoon chili powder

¼ teaspoon cayenne pepper

4 eggs

6 flour tortillas

½ cup (58 g) shredded low-fat cheddar cheese

—
Yield: 6 servings

Brown sausage in frying pan; add chopped onion, chili powder, and cayenne pepper. Cook for 10 minutes. Drain and discard any fat. Add eggs. Stir until eggs are set. Spoon mixture into center of warmed tortilla, top with shredded cheese, and roll up tortilla.

NUTRITIONAL ANALYSIS

EACH WITH: 52 g water; 11 g protein; 10 g total fat; 4 g saturated fat; 3 g monounsaturated fat; 2 g polyunsaturated fat; 18 g carb; 1 g fiber; 1 g sugar; 166 mg phosphorus; 101 mg calcium; 2 mg iron; 485 mg sodium; 157 mg potassium; 177 IU vitamin A; 13 mg vitamin C; 25 mg cholesterol

Basque Breakfast Skillet

201 CALORIES (43% FROM FAT, 25% FROM PROTEIN, 32% FROM CARB)

This is an entire breakfast in a pan.

4 slices bacon

2 potatoes, shredded

2 teaspoons sliced green onion (tops)

1 tablespoon (4 g) snipped parsley

⅛ teaspoon crushed dried thyme

¾ teaspoon salt

¼ teaspoon pepper

4 large eggs

½ cup (120 ml) milk

—

Yield: 4 servings

Fry the bacon in a heavy skillet over medium-high heat until crisp. Remove the bacon and crumble. Pour off all but 2 tablespoons (30 ml) of the drippings. Return the skillet to the stove and reduce heat to low. Add the potatoes, onion, parsley, thyme, salt, and pepper to the skillet, cover, and cook until the potatoes are just tender (about 8 minutes), stirring occasionally. Beat together the eggs and milk and pour over the potato mixture. Cover and continue cooking until the mixture is set to your liking (about 10 minutes). Serve with sour cream and the bacon bits sprinkled over the top. (A splash of Tabasco will get your morning off on the right foot too!)

NUTRITIONAL ANALYSIS

EACH WITH: 125 g water; 13 g protein; 10 g total fat; 3 g saturated fat; 4 g monounsaturated fat; 1 g polyunsaturated fat; 16 g carb; 1 g fiber; 3 g sugar; 215 mg phosphorus; 81 mg calcium; 2 mg iron; 727 mg sodium; 444 mg potassium; 370 IU vitamin A; 11 mg vitamin C; 248 mg cholesterol

Italian Breakfast Casserole

440 CALORIES (70% FROM FAT, 24% FROM PROTEIN, 6% FROM CARB)

I probably should say "Italian flavored." Something like this has most likely never been seen in Italy, but it seemed like a good idea when I created it. And everyone liked it, so I'm sure we'll have it again.

1 pound (455 g) Italian sausage, casings removed

1 tablespoon (14 g) butter

4 ounces (115 g) mushrooms, sliced

1 cup (160 g) red onion, chopped

12 eggs, beaten

1 cup (235 ml) milk

8 ounces (115 g) mozzarella cheese, shredded

1 cup (180 g) tomatoes, peeled and chopped

½ teaspoon freshly ground pepper

½ teaspoon oregano, crumbled

—
Yield: 8 servings

Sauté crumbled sausage until no longer pink. Drain and put aside in bowl. Sauté onion and mushrooms in butter until soft but not brown. Stir into sausage. Blend in remaining ingredients and mix well. Pour into greased 9 × 13-inch (23 × 33 cm) pan and bake at 400°F (200°C, or gas mark 6) for 30 to 35 minutes or until knife inserted in center comes out clean.

NUTRITIONAL ANALYSIS

EACH WITH: 183 g water; 27 g Protein; 34 g total fat; 14 g saturated fat; 14 g monounsaturated fat; 4 g polyunsaturated fat; 6 g carb; 1 g fiber; 4 g sugar; 395 mg phosphorous; 244 mg calcium; 3 mg iron; 736 mg sodium; 444 mg potassium; 829 IU vitamin A; 197 mg ATE vitamin E; 8 mg vitamin C; 425 mg cholesterol

Hash Brown Omelet

236 CALORIES (52% FROM FAT, 24% FROM PROTEIN, 24% FROM CARB)

This is more like a frittata than an omelet really. The potatoes and veggies are browned, and then eggs are poured over and cooked until they are set without stirring.

4 slices bacon

2 cups (420 g) frozen hash brown potatoes

¼ cup (40 g) onion, chopped

¼ cup (38 g) green pepper, chopped

4 eggs

¼ cup (60 ml) skim milk

1 cup (115 g) cheddar, shredded

¼ teaspoon pepper

—
Yield: 6 servings

In a 10 or 12-inch (25 or 30 cm) skillet, cook bacon until crisp. Leave some drippings and remove bacon. Brown potatoes, onion, and green pepper and pat down into bottom of pan. Blend eggs, milk, and pepper and pour over potatoes. Top with cheese and crumbled bacon. Cover and cook over low heat until egg is set.

NUTRITIONAL ANALYSIS

EACH WITH: 113 g water; 14 g Protein; 14 g total fat; 7 g saturated fat; 4 g monounsaturated fat; 1 g polyunsaturated fat; 14 g carb; 1 g fiber; 1 g sugar; 259 mg phosphorous; 201 mg calcium; 2 mg iron; 333 mg sodium; 338 mg potassium; 448 IU vitamin A; 115 mg ATE vitamin E; 11 mg vitamin C; 187 mg cholesterol

TIP

Make it even easier on yourself and get the frozen O'Brien potatoes, which have the onions and peppers already added.

Veggie Frittata

140 CALORIES (26% FROM FAT, 51% FROM PROTEIN, 22% FROM CARB)

A frittata is an Italian-style omelet with the filling mixed in with the eggs. It's cooked without turning, and then the top is set under the broiler. This version does not have any of the meat and potatoes that they often have, providing you with a filling weekend breakfast low in sodium, fat, and carbohydrates.

½ cup (75 g) chopped red bell pepper

½ cup (80 g) chopped onion

1 cup (71 g) broccoli florets

8 ounces (225 g) sliced mushrooms

1 cup (113 g) sliced zucchini

6 eggs

1 tablespoon (4 g) parsley

¼ teaspoon black pepper

2 ounces (55 g) Swiss cheese, shredded

—
Yield: 4 servings

Coat a large ovenproof skillet with nonstick vegetable oil spray. Stir-fry the bell pepper, onion, and broccoli until crisp-tender. Add the mushrooms and zucchini and stir-fry 1 to 2 minutes more. Stir together the eggs, parsley, and black pepper and pour over vegetable mixture, spreading to cover. Cover and cook over medium heat 10 to 12 minutes or until eggs are nearly set. Sprinkle cheese over top. Place the skillet under broiler until eggs are set and cheese is melted.

NUTRITIONAL ANALYSIS

EACH WITH: 220 g water; 18 g protein; 4 g total fat; 1 g saturated fat; 1 g monounsaturated fat; 2 g polyunsaturated fat; 8 g carb; 2 g fiber; 4 g sugar; 283 mg phosphorus; 209 mg calcium; 3 mg iron; 216 mg sodium; 721 mg potassium; 1,618 IU vitamin A; 50 mg vitamin C; 66 mg cholesterol

Cottage Cheese Pancakes

270 CALORIES (35% FROM FAT, 23% FROM PROTEIN, 42% FROM CARB)

These pancakes are lighter than most, thanks to the addition of cottage cheese.

3 eggs

¼ cup (6 g) Splenda

¼ teaspoon salt

1 cup (225 g) cottage cheese

¼ cup (60 ml) skim milk

1 cup (125 g) flour

2 tablespoons (28 g) butter, melted

—

Yield: 4 servings

Beat the eggs with Splenda and salt. Add cottage cheese and milk and beat well. Gradually add flour and beat until smooth. Stir in melted butter. Pour spoonfuls on greased griddle. Turn when lightly browned and brown on other side.

NUTRITIONAL ANALYSIS

EACH WITH: 80 g water; 15 g Protein; 10 g total fat; 5 g saturated fat; 3 g monounsaturated fat; 1 g polyunsaturated fat; 28 g carb; 1 g fiber; 4 g sugar; 169 mg phosphorous; 59 mg calcium; 2 mg iron; 111 mg sodium; 127 mg potassium; 424 IU vitamin A; 119 mg ATE vitamin E; 0 mg vitamin C; 196 mg cholesterol

Apple and Banana Fritters

212 CALORIES (23% FROM FAT, 13% FROM PROTEIN, 64% FROM CARB)

A search for something for breakfast that would use up some overripe bananas was rewarded with this recipe. They are incredibly light and very tasty.

1 cup (120 g) whole wheat pastry flour

1 tablespoon (1½ g) sugar substitute, such as Splenda

1 tablespoon (14 g) baking powder

½ cup (120 ml) skim milk

1 egg

1 tablespoon (15 ml) canola oil

½ cup (75 g) chopped banana

½ cup (63 g) chopped apple

½ teaspoon nutmeg

—

Yield: 4 servings

Stir together flour, sugar substitute, and baking powder. Combine the milk, egg, and oil. Add banana, apple, and nutmeg. Stir into dry ingredients, stirring until just moistened. Drop by tablespoonfuls into hot oil. Fry for 2 to 3 minutes on a side until golden brown. Drain on paper towels before serving.

NUTRITIONAL ANALYSIS

EACH WITH: 74 g water; 7 g protein; 6 g total fat; 1 g saturated fat; 3 g monounsaturated fat; 1 g polyunsaturated fat; 36 g carb; 5 g fiber; 8 g sugar; 249 mg phosphorus; 267 mg calcium; 2 mg iron; 405 mg sodium; 311 mg potassium; 157 IU vitamin A; 3 mg vitamin C; 60 mg cholesterol

Orange Smoothie

414 CALORIES (7% FROM FAT, 14% FROM PROTEIN, 79% FROM CARB)

Buttermilk and orange juice concentrate provide the flavor here. And a great flavor it is.

1½ cup (355 ml) buttermilk

⅓ cup (83 g) orange juice concentrate

2 tablespoons (30 g) brown sugar

1 teaspoon vanilla

2 ice cubes

—

Yield: 1 serving

In a blender container, combine buttermilk, orange juice concentrate, brown sugar, and vanilla. Cover and blend until smooth. With blender running, add ice cubes one at a time, through opening in lid. Blend until smooth and frothy.

NUTRITIONAL ANALYSIS

EACH WITH: 389 g water; 14 g Protein; 3 g total fat; 2 g saturated fat; 1 g monounsaturated fat; 0 g polyunsaturated fat; 81 g carb; 1 g fiber; 80 g sugar; 387 mg phosphorous; 480 mg calcium; 1 mg iron; 400 mg sodium; 1295 mg potassium; 454 IU vitamin A; 26 mg ATE vitamin E; 134 mg vitamin C; 15 mg cholesterol

Mixed Fruit Smoothie

485 CALORIES (7% FROM FAT,
10% FROM PROTEIN, 83% FROM CARB)

Smoothies make a quick and easy breakfast, and they are packed with nutrition.

2 cups (460 g) low-fat peach yogurt

1 cup (145 g) blueberries

2 cups (300 g) sliced banana

—

Yield: 2 servings

Mix all ingredients in a blender and then serve.

NUTRITIONAL ANALYSIS

EACH WITH: 415 g water; 13 g protein; 4 g total fat;
2 g saturated fat; 1 g monounsaturated fat;
0 g polyunsaturated fat; 108 g carb; 8 g fiber;
81 g sugar; 325 mg phosphorus; 354 mg calcium;
1 mg iron; 133 mg sodium; 1,296 mg potassium;
282 IU vitamin A; 28 mg vitamin C; 12 mg cholesterol

Pineapple Boats

460 CALORIES (25% FROM FAT,
19% FROM PROTEIN, 56% FROM CARB)

Are you looking for a breakfast meal that's fancy enough to serve guests but doesn't take a long time to fix? These pineapple boats will definitely do the trick.

2 pineapples

1 cup (150 g) seedless green grapes

2 cups (450 g) bananas, sliced

2 tablespoons (30 g) brown sugar

1 teaspoon poppy seeds

½ pound (225 g) ham, thinly sliced

¼ pound (115 g) Swiss cheese, cubed

—

Yield: 4 servings

Slice pineapple lengthwise in half, crown to stem. Leave leafy crown on. Remove tough core. Loosen fruit by cutting to rind; cut in bite size pieces. Place in large bowl. Peel bananas; slice. Cut grapes in half and add to pineapple. Toss with brown sugar and poppy seeds. Line pineapple shells with ham. Spoon fruit mixture on top. Top with cheese.

NUTRITIONAL ANALYSIS

EACH WITH: 356 g water; 23 g Protein; 14 g total fat;
7 g saturated fat; 4 g monounsaturated fat;
1 g polyunsaturated fat; 68 g carb; 7 g fiber;
46 g sugar; 350 mg phosphorous; 332 mg calcium;
2 mg iron; 616 mg sodium; 977 mg potassium;
459 IU vitamin A; 60 mg ATE vitamin E;
96 mg vitamin C; 49 mg cholesterol

CHAPTER 5

Main Dishes: Vegetarian

Vegetarian meals are a great way to up the number of vegetable servings you are eating and get some high-quality protein without either the high-GI carbs or the fat that meat dishes often contain. We have here a selection of quiches and omelets, tofu and portobello mushroom dishes, and soups that will satisfy even the people who think they have to have meat at every meal.

Onion Pie

268 CALORIES (52% FROM FAT, 9% FROM PROTEIN, 39% FROM CARB)

There's an old saying around our house that you can never have too many onions, so you can probably guess that this pie is popular.

2 tablespoons (30 ml) olive oil

3 cups (480 g) onions, finely diced

1 cup (235 ml) skim milk

8 ounces (225 g) tofu, crushed by hand

¼ teaspoon black pepper

⅛ teaspoon nutmeg

2 tablespoons (16 g) flour

1 pie crust

—
Yield: 6 servings

Sauté onions in oil until translucent and mostly soft. Blend the milk, tofu, pepper, nutmeg, and flour until smooth. Then combine the onions and the milk mixture. Pour into the prepared pie shell. Bake in a preheated oven at 350°F (180°C, or gas mark 4) for about 30 minutes.

NUTRITIONAL ANALYSIS

EACH WITH: 149 g water; 6 g Protein; 16 g total fat; 3 g saturated fat; 8 g monounsaturated fat; 4 g polyunsaturated fat; 26 g carb; 3 g fiber; 6 g sugar; 110 mg phosphorous; 85 mg calcium; 1 mg iron; 27 mg sodium; 272 mg potassium; 85 IU vitamin A; 25 mg ATE vitamin E; 6 mg vitamin C; 1 mg cholesterol

Eggplant Lasagna

192 CALORIES (36% FROM FAT, 21% FROM PROTEIN, 43% FROM CARB)

This is truly vegetarian version of lasagna with a flavor that will please even the meat lovers in your family.

1 medium eggplant

2 tablespoons (30 ml) lemon juice

¼ cup (31 g) flour

¼ cup (35 g) cornmeal

½ teaspoon oregano

½ teaspoon garlic powder

⅛ teaspoon black pepper

2 tablespoons (30 ml) oil

FILLING

1½ pounds (680 g) firm tofu

¼ cup (60 ml) lemon juice

2 teaspoons (2.8 g) dried basil

1 garlic clove

1½ cup (368 g) tomato sauce

—
Yield: 6 servings

Wash, peel, and slice eggplant into ¼-inch (½ cm) pieces. Spread slices out on racks or paper towels and then sprinkle with lemon juice. Let stand 5 to 10 minutes and then wipe off with paper towels. While eggplant is standing, mix flour, cornmeal, oregano, garlic powder, and black pepper together in a bowl. Preheat oven to 350°F (180°C, or gas mark 4). Dredge eggplant slices in flour-cornmeal mix. Lay on cookie sheet spread with the oil. Oven-fry slices for 8 to 10 minutes on each side or until golden brown. While the eggplant slices are baking, prepare the tofu filling. Process the tofu, lemon juice, basil, and garlic in food processor to a fine grainy texture like ricotta cheese. Cover bottom of 8 × 8-inch (20 × 20 cm) pan with ⅓ of the tomato sauce. Use half the oven fried eggplant slices to cover the bottom of the pan. Then spread the tofu filling over, reserving ½ cup (125 g) for the top. Next, cover the tofu filling with the rest of the eggplant slices and pour the remaining tomato sauce over the top. Arrange reserved tofu mix in small dollops over the top. Bake about 45 minutes or until dollops are slightly browned.

NUTRITIONAL ANALYSIS

EACH WITH: 241 g water; 11 g Protein; 8 g total fat; 1 g saturated fat; 2 g monounsaturated fat; 4 g polyunsaturated fat; 21 g carb; 4 g fiber; 6 g sugar; 153 mg phosphorous; 60 mg calcium; 3 mg iron; 364 mg sodium; 645 mg potassium; 279 IU vitamin A; 0 mg ATE vitamin E; 13 mg vitamin C; 0 mg cholesterol

Vegetable "Lasagna"

158 CALORIES (32% FROM FAT, 25% FROM PROTEIN, 43% FROM CARB)

You could use this as a side dish with something like a grilled chicken breast or just serve it as a vegetarian main dish. I used a George Foreman grill to grill the vegetables, but you could also use a regular grill or roast them in the oven.

4 cups (452 g) zucchini, sliced lengthwise

1 eggplant, sliced

8 ounces (225 g) mushrooms, sliced

1 onion, sliced

2 cups (500 g) spaghetti sauce

1 cup (115 g) shredded mozzarella cheese

—
Yield: 6 servings

Slice vegetables and coat with olive oil spray. Grill until crisp-tender. Place a small amount of sauce in an 8 × 12-inch (20 × 30 cm) baking dish. Layer zucchini, eggplant, more sauce, onion and mushroom, sauce, eggplant, and zucchini. Top with remaining sauce and sprinkle with cheese. Bake at 400°F (200°C, gas mark 6) until cheese is melted and starts to brown, about 15 minutes.

NUTRITIONAL ANALYSIS

285 g water; 10 g protein; 6 g total fat; 3 g saturated fat; 2 g mono-unsaturated fat; 1 g polyunsaturated fat; 18 g carb; 6 g fiber; 10 g sugar; 204 mg calcium; 1 mg iron; 40 mg sodium; 807 mg potassium; 912 IU vitamin A; 25 mg vitamin C; 12 mg cholesterol

Spinach Rolls

245 CALORIES (54% FROM FAT, 11% FROM PROTEIN, 35% FROM CARB)

There's something special about anything that has phyllo pastry in it and these rolls are no exception. They are a bit of work to assemble, but they are worth the effort.

2 pounds (900 g) spinach

1 cup (160 g) onion, chopped

1 cup (104 g) leek, chopped

1 cup (100 g) green onion, sliced

⅓ cup (80 ml) olive oil

½ cup (30 g) chopped fresh parsley

3 teaspoons (4 g) chopped fresh dill

¼ teaspoon ground nutmeg

¼ teaspoon freshly ground black pepper

8 phyllo pastry sheets

2 tablespoons (30 ml) olive oil

—

Yield: 8 servings

Wash spinach well and cut off any coarse stems. Chop coarsely and put into a large pan. Cover and place over heat for 7 to 8 minutes, shaking pan now and then or turning spinach with a fork. Heat just long enough to wilt spinach so that juices can run out freely. Drain well in colander, pressing occasionally with a spoon. Gently fry onions in olive oil for 10 minutes; add chopped leek and green onions and fry gently for 5 minutes until transparent. Place well-drained spinach in a mixing bowl and add oil and onion mixture, herbs, nutmeg, and pepper. Blend thoroughly. Place a sheet of phyllo pastry on work surface and brush lightly with olive oil. Top with 3 more sheets of pastry, brushing each with oil. Brush top layer lightly with oil and place half the spinach mixture along the length of the pastry towards one edge and leaving 1½ inches (3½ cm) clear on each side. Fold bottom edge of pastry over filling, roll once, fold in sides, and then roll up. Place a hand at each end of roll and push it in gently. Repeat with remaining pastry and filling. Place rolls in an oiled baking dish, leaving space between rolls. Brush tops lightly with oil and bake in a moderate oven for 30 minutes until golden. Serve hot, cut into portions.

NUTRITIONAL ANALYSIS

EACH WITH: 149 g water; 7 g Protein; 16 g total fat; 3 g saturated fat; 10 g monounsaturated fat; 2 g polyunsaturated fat; 23 g carb; 6 g fiber; 3 g sugar; 98 mg phosphorous; 216 mg calcium; 4 mg iron; 211 mg sodium; 489 mg potassium; 14331 IU vitamin A; 0 mg ATE vitamin E; 13 mg vitamin C; 0 mg cholesterol

Stuffed Portobellos

75 CALORIES (40% FROM FAT, 29% FROM PROTEIN, 32% FROM CARB)

We recently discovered the joys of portobello mushrooms. This has become one of our favorite recipes.

⅔ cup (120 g) chopped plum tomato

2 ounces (55 g) part-skim mozzarella cheese, shredded

1 teaspoon olive oil, divided

½ teaspoon fresh rosemary

⅛ teaspoon black pepper, coarse ground

¼ teaspoon crushed garlic

4 portobello mushroom caps, about 4 to 5 inches (10 to 13 cm)

2 tablespoons (30 ml) lemon juice

2 teaspoons (2.6 g) fresh parsley

—

Yield: 4 servings

Prepare grill. Combine the tomato, cheese, ½ teaspoon oil, rosemary, pepper, and garlic in a small bowl. Remove brown gills from the undersides of mushroom caps using a spoon and discard gills. Remove stems and discard. Combine remaining ½ teaspoon oil and lemon juice in a small bowl. Brush over both sides of mushroom caps. Place the mushroom caps, stem sides down, on grill rack coated with nonstick vegetable oil spray and grill for 5 minutes on each side or until soft. Spoon ¼ cup tomato mixture into each mushroom cap. Cover and grill 3 minutes or until cheese is melted. Sprinkle with parsley.

NUTRITIONAL ANALYSIS

EACH WITH: 115 g water; 6 g protein; 4 g total fat; 2 g saturated fat; 1 g monounsaturated fat; 0 g polyunsaturated fat; 6 g carb; 2 g fiber; 3 g sugar; 181 mg phosphorus; 122 mg calcium; 1 mg iron; 95 mg sodium; 490 mg potassium; 331 IU vitamin A; 8 mg vitamin C; 9 mg cholesterol

Vegetable Burgers

212 CALORIES (24% FROM FAT, 24% FROM PROTEIN, 51% FROM CARB)

Many people think of veggie burgers as being dry and tasteless. These will change their minds.

1 pound (455 g) tofu, mashed

1 cup (80 g) quick cooking oats

½ cup (56 g) wheat germ

1 cup (160 g) onion,
finely minced

2 tablespoons (30 ml)
Reduced-Sodium Soy Sauce
(see chapter 2)

½ teaspoon basil

½ teaspoon oregano

½ teaspoon garlic powder

⅛ teaspoon black pepper

—
Yield: 4 servings

Mix ingredients together. Knead for a few minutes. Shape into six patties. Oven fry on cookie sheet sprayed with nonstick oil spray at 325°F (170°C, or gas mark 3) for 25 minutes.

NUTRITIONAL ANALYSIS

EACH WITH: 139 g water; 13 g Protein; 6 g total fat; 1 g saturated fat; 1 g monounsaturated fat; 3 g polyunsaturated fat; 28 g carb; 5 g fiber; 5 g sugar; 342 mg phosphorous; 66 mg calcium; 3 mg iron; 9 mg sodium; 477 mg potassium; 32 IU vitamin A; 0 mg ATE vitamin E; 4 mg vitamin C; 0 mg cholesterol

Black Bean Quesadillas

457 CALORIES (30% FROM FAT, 19% FROM PROTEIN, 51% FROM CARB)

I usually add a bit more cilantro because I like the flavor (and I'm the cook so I can). Use mild or hot salsa according to your own taste.

15 ounces (420 g) black beans, drained

¼ cup (45 g) chopped tomato

3 tablespoons (4 g) chopped cilantro

12 black olives, pitted, sliced

8 whole wheat tortillas, 6-inch (15 cm)

4 ounces (58 g) pepper jack cheese, shredded

1 cup (30 g) spinach leaves, shredded

4 tablespoons (65 g) salsa

—
Yield: 4 servings

Mash beans. Stir in tomato, cilantro, and olives. Spread evenly onto 4 tortillas. Sprinkle with cheese, spinach, and salsa. Top with remaining tortillas. Preheat oven to 350°F (180°C, or gas mark 4). Bake tortillas on ungreased cookie sheet for 12 minutes. Cut into wedges and serve.

NUTRITIONAL ANALYSIS

EACH WITH: 142 g water; 22 g Protein; 15 g total fat; 7 g saturated fat; 6 g monounsaturated fat; 2 g polyunsaturated fat; 59 g carb; 12 g fiber; 2 g sugar; 362 mg phosphorous; 344 mg calcium; 5 mg iron; 696 mg sodium; 618 mg potassium; 1238 IU vitamin A; 54 mg ATE vitamin E; 4 mg vitamin C; 25 mg cholesterol

Beans and Barley

487 CALORIES (6% FROM FAT, 26% FROM PROTEIN, 68% FROM CARB)

This hearty main dish cooks in the slow cooker while you are gone.

1 cup (215 g) white beans, uncooked

1 cup (193 g) pinto beans, uncooked

¾ cup (120 g) onion, chopped

1 cup (130 g) carrot, chopped

½ cup (35 g) mushrooms, chopped

4 cups (940 g) low-sodium vegetable broth

½ teaspoon prepared mustard

2 tablespoons (8 g) fresh parsley, minced

½ cup (113 g) split peas, dried

¼ cup (50 g) pearl barley

¼ cup (48 g) lentils, dried

—

Yield: 4 servings

Soak white beans and pinto beans overnight. Sauté onion, mushrooms, and carrots in 1 tablespoon (15 ml) of vegetable stock until tender. To sautéed vegetables, add drained beans, vegetable stock, mustard, and parsley. Bring to boil. Reduce heat, cover, and simmer 45 minutes. Add split peas, lentils, and barley. Transfer all ingredients to a big slow cooker set on low for 12 to 14 hours.

NUTRITIONAL ANALYSIS

EACH WITH: 337 g water; 33 g Protein; 3 g total fat; 1 g saturated fat; 1 g monounsaturated fat; 1 g polyunsaturated fat; 84 g carb; 22 g fiber; 6 g sugar; 529 mg phosphorous; 279 mg calcium; 10 mg iron; 181 mg sodium; 2160 mg potassium; 5554 IU vitamin A; 2 mg ATE vitamin E; 10 mg vitamin C; 0 mg cholesterol

Mexican Vegetable Casserole

241 CALORIES (53% FROM FAT, 15% FROM PROTEIN, 32% FROM CARB)

This squash casserole gets a Mexican makeover with the addition of chilies and cheese.
This makes a great side dish with simple grilled beef or chicken rubbed with Mexican spices.

4 cups (480 g) zucchini, sliced

1 cup (160 g) onion, chopped

3 tablespoons (45 ml) olive oil

2 cloves garlic

4 ounces (115 g) chopped green chilies

16 ounces (455 g) frozen corn

1 cup (120 g) cheddar, grated

—

Yield: 6 servings

Sauté squash and onion in oil until barely tender. Add garlic, chilies, corn, and cheese; mix well. Put in buttered 1-quart (1 L) casserole and bake at 400°F (200°C, or gas mark 6) for 20 minutes.

NUTRITIONAL ANALYSIS

EACH WITH: 185 g water; 9 g Protein; 15 g total fat; 6 g saturated fat; 7 g monounsaturated fat; 1 g polyunsaturated fat; 21 g carb; 4 g fiber; 5 g sugar; 221 mg phosphorous; 186 mg calcium; 1 mg iron; 232 mg sodium; 503 mg potassium; 567 IU vitamin A; 57 mg ATE vitamin E; 28 mg vitamin C; 23 mg cholesterol

Curried Lentil Stew

112 CALORIES (29% FROM FAT, 13% FROM PROTEIN, 58% FROM CARB)

We don't have lentils as often as we probably should. When I make something like this tasty stew, I wonder why.

2 tablespoons (30 ml) olive oil

1 cup (160 g) onion, chopped

2 garlic cloves, chopped

1 medium potato, diced

½ cup (65 g) carrot, sliced

½ cup (75 g) green bell peppers, diced

1 tablespoon (6 g) coriander

1 teaspoon cumin

1 teaspoon ginger

1 teaspoon turmeric

1 cup (192 g) lentils

2 cups (475 ml) water

2 tablespoons (32 g) tomato paste

—

Yield: 8 servings

In a large pot, heat oil. Fry onion and garlic for a couple of minutes. Add potatoes, carrots and bell pepper and continue to fry for a few more minutes, stirring occasionally. Add spices and stir-fry for a couple of seconds. Add lentils and tomato paste, stir quickly, and add water. Cover, raise heat and bring to a boil. Reduce heat and simmer gently for 30 minutes. Check the water levels and lentil consistency. Cook for another 15 minutes if lentils are not cooked. Remove from heat and let cool slightly. The mixture should be moist but not overly thin.

NUTRITIONAL ANALYSIS

EACH WITH: 142 g water; 4 g Protein; 4 g total fat; 1 g saturated fat; 3 g monounsaturated fat; 0 g polyunsaturated fat; 17 g carb; 4 g fiber; 3 g sugar; 89 mg phosphorous; 25 mg calcium; 2 mg iron; 47 mg sodium; 433 mg potassium; 1465 IU vitamin A; 0 mg ATE vitamin E; 17 mg vitamin C; 0 mg cholesterol

Italian Chickpea Sauce

196 CALORIES (23% FROM FAT, 16% FROM PROTEIN, 61% FROM CARB)

Can a pasta sauce be made with chickpeas? Yes, and you won't believe how good it is until you try it.

1½ cup (360 g) dried chick peas, soaked

1 tablespoon (15 ml) olive oil

¾ cup (120 g) onion, chopped

2 garlic cloves, crushed

14 ounces (400 g) no-salt-added tomatoes, chopped

6 ounces (170 g) no-salt-added tomato paste

1 teaspoon basil

1 teaspoon oregano

1 dash cinnamon

2 tablespoons (8 g) fresh parsley

—
Yield: 4 servings

Rinse chickpeas, place in fresh water, and cook for 50 minutes or until tender. Heat oil in large pot and sauté onions and garlic for a few minutes. Add the tomatoes and tomato paste. Bring to a boil, lower heat, and add the rest of the ingredients. Simmer for about 10 minutes or until the sauce has thickened.

NUTRITIONAL ANALYSIS

EACH WITH: 190 g water; 8 g Protein; 5 g total fat; 1 g saturated fat; 3 g monounsaturated fat; 1 g polyunsaturated fat; 32 g carb; 8 g fiber; 12 g sugar; 169 mg phosphorous; 93 mg calcium; 4 mg iron; 61 mg sodium; 861 mg potassium; 973 IU vitamin A; 0 mg ATE vitamin E; 24 mg vitamin C; 0 mg cholesterol

Quick Black Bean and Corn Chili

369 CALORIES (31% FROM FAT, 22% FROM PROTEIN, 46% FROM CARB)

Canned sauce and beans make this chili one of the quickest meals you'll find. But don't let that fool you; the flavor is still full and well developed.

16 ounces (455 g) picante sauce

15 ounces (420 g) black beans, undrained

8 ounces (225 g) no-salt-added tomato sauce

1 cup (164 g) frozen corn

½ teaspoon cumin

1 cup (115 g) cheddar, shredded

2 tablespoons (30 g) sour cream

—
Yield: 4 servings

In medium saucepan, combine picante sauce, beans, tomato sauce, corn, and cumin. Bring to boil; reduce heat; simmer 5 minutes. Divide among serving bowls; top with cheese and sour cream.

NUTRITIONAL ANALYSIS

EACH WITH: 274 g water; 21 g Protein; 13 g total fat; 8 g saturated fat; 4 g monounsaturated fat; 1 g polyunsaturated fat; 44 g carb; 11 g fiber; 7 g sugar; 368 mg phosphorous; 303 mg calcium; 3 mg iron; 665 mg sodium; 695 mg potassium; 1035 IU vitamin A; 93 mg ATE vitamin E; 16 mg vitamin C; 38 mg cholesterol

Greek Vegetable Casserole

582 CALORIES (55% FROM FAT, 6% FROM PROTEIN, 39% FROM CARB)

This Mediterranean vegetable casserole is almost a meal in itself. It goes very well with fish or chicken.

1 eggplant

2 pounds (900 g) zucchini

4 medium potatoes

1 green bell pepper

1 red bell pepper

2 small onions

1 cup (235 ml) olive oil

4 medium tomatoes

2 cloves garlic

1 teaspoon sugar

Black pepper, to taste

—

Yield: 6 servings

Prepare the vegetables: Cut the eggplant, zucchini, and potatoes in bite sized chunks (do not peel the zucchini or the eggplant). Remove the stems and seeds from the peppers and slice them into strips. Peel and slice the onions. Dice the tomatoes. Sauté the vegetables except the tomatoes in the olive oil in small batches. Sauté each batch for 2 or 3 minutes and then remove from the pan, trying to drain some of the oil so that enough oil is left for the next batch. Place the sautéed vegetables in a baking dish and toss them briefly. Add the tomatoes into the pan and sauté for a couple of minutes. Crush the garlic and add to the tomatoes. Add the sugar and pepper to taste and simmer for another minute. Pour the tomato sauce on top of the vegetables.

NUTRITIONAL ANALYSIS

PER SERVING: 589 g water; 9 g Protein; 37 g total fat; 5 g saturated fat; 26 g monounsaturated fat; 4 g polyunsaturated fat; 60 g carb; 11 g fiber; 10 g sugar; 273 mg phosphorous; 71 mg calcium; 3 mg iron; 45 mg sodium; 2078 mg potassium; 1917 IU vitamin A; 0 mg ATE vitamin E; 132 mg vitamin C; 0 mg cholesterol

CHAPTER 6

Main Dishes: Fish and Seafood

Like vegetarian meals, fish and seafood are low in fat and lend themselves to dishes that feature vegetables and not the higher-GI carbohydrates. Tuna and salmon feature prominently here, but there are also lots of other fish and seafood—all in a variety of flavors from Maryland to Italy to Southeast Asia.

Grilled Salmon Fillets

334 CALORIES (45% FROM FAT, 37% FROM PROTEIN, 18% FROM CARB)

You can use a whole salmon fillet for this recipe. It makes an impressive display, but it can be difficult to turn. I usually cut the fillet into serving-size pieces, but then you need to be careful not to overcook them and dry them out. The sweetness of the sauce goes well with the salmon.

¼ cup (60 g) brown sugar

2 tablespoons (30 ml)
cider vinegar

2 tablespoons (40 g) honey

¼ teaspoon liquid smoke

¼ teaspoon black pepper

¼ teaspoon crushed garlic

2 pounds (900 g) salmon fillets

—
Yield: 6 servings

Preheat the grill. In a small mixing bowl, combine sauce ingredients. Mix well. Brush one side of the salmon with the basting sauce and then place the salmon (basted side down) on the grill. When the salmon is half finished cooking, baste the top portion of the salmon and flip the fillet so the fresh basting sauce is on the grill. When the fish is almost finished cooking, apply the basting sauce and flip the salmon again. Baste and flip the salmon once more and serve. Be careful not to overcook the salmon, as it will lose its juices and flavor if cooked too long.

NUTRITIONAL ANALYSIS

EACH WITH: 110 g water; 30 g protein; 16 g total fat; 3 g saturated fat; 6 g monounsaturated fat; 6 g polyunsaturated fat; 15 g carb; 0 g fiber; 15 g sugar; 355 mg phosphorus; 27 mg calcium; 1 mg iron; 93 mg sodium; 587 mg potassium; 76 IU vitamin A; 6 mg vitamin C; 89 mg cholesterol

Grilled Tuna with Honey Mustard

275 CALORIES (53% FROM FAT, 40% FROM PROTEIN, 7% FROM CARB)

These tuna steaks can be grilled or broiled. If it's not good weather for outdoor grilling, they also work well on a contact grill like the George Foreman models.

⅓ cup (80 ml) red wine vinegar

1 tablespoon (11 g) spicy brown mustard

1 tablespoon (20 g) honey

3 tablespoons (45 ml) extra virgin olive oil

1 pound (455 g) tuna steaks

—
Yield: 4 servings

Combine the first 4 ingredients in a jar or covered container; shake to mix well. Put tuna in a food storage bag; add the mustard mixture. Seal the bag and let marinate for about 20 minutes. Heat the grill. Remove the tuna from the marinade and pour the marinade in a small saucepan. Bring marinade to a boil; remove from heat and set aside. Grill the tuna over high heat for about 2 minutes on each side or until done as desired. Drizzle with the hot marinade.

NUTRITIONAL ANALYSIS

EACH WITH: 100 g water; 27 g protein; 16 g total fat; 3 g saturated fat; 9 g monounsaturated fat; 3 g polyunsaturated fat; 5 g carb; 0 g fiber; 4 g sugar; 294 mg phosphorus; 13 mg calcium; 1 mg iron; 89 mg sodium; 302 mg potassium; 2,478 IU vitamin A; 0 mg vitamin C; 43 mg cholesterol

Tuna Steaks

247 CALORIES (65% FROM FAT, 33% FROM PROTEIN, 3% FROM CARB)

If you get them on sale, tuna steaks are one of the cheaper fish products you can buy. The key to cooking them is not to overcook them and dry them out. It's all right for them to be medium or even medium rare. Soaking them in a simple marinade also helps to keep them moist and flavorful.

6 ounces (170 g) tuna steaks

2 tablespoons (30 ml) olive oil

2 tablespoons (30 ml) lemon juice

½ teaspoon black pepper, fresh ground

—

Yield: 2 servings

Combine the olive oil and lemon juice. Marinate the steaks in the mixture at least 30 minutes, turning occasionally. Heat a skillet over high heat. Add the steaks and cook 2 minutes. Sprinkle with pepper, turn over, and cook 2 minutes longer.

NUTRITIONAL ANALYSIS

EACH WITH: 72 g water; 20 g protein; 18 g total fat; 3 g saturated fat; 11 g monounsaturated fat; 3 g polyunsaturated fat; 2 g carb; 0 g fiber; 0 g sugar; 10 mg calcium; 1 mg iron; 34 mg sodium; 240 mg potassium; 1,861 IU vitamin A; 7 mg vitamin C; 32 mg cholesterol

Parmesan Crusted Catfish

412 CALORIES (60% FROM FAT, 30% FROM PROTEIN, 10% FROM CARB)

Catfish is one of our favorite fish and this crunchy presentation is one of our favorite ways to prepare it. It's perfect with just a steamed fresh vegetable.

8 catfish fillets

1 cup (115 g) bread crumbs

¾ cup (75 g) parmesan cheese, grated

¼ cup (15 g) fresh parsley, chopped

1 teaspoon paprika

½ teaspoon oregano

¼ teaspoon basil

½ teaspoon pepper

½ cup (112 g) melted butter

—

Yield: 8 servings

Pat fish dry. Combine bread crumbs, cheese, and seasonings; stir well. Dip catfish in butter and roll each in crumb mixture. Arrange fish in well-greased 13 × 9 × 2-inch (33 × 23 × 5 cm) baking dish. Bake at 375°F (190°C, or gas mark 4) about 25 minutes or until fish flakes easily when tested with a fork.

NUTRITIONAL ANALYSIS

EACH WITH: 127 g water; 30 g Protein; 27 g total fat; 12 g saturated fat; 10 g monounsaturated fat; 3 g polyunsaturated fat; 10 g carb; 1 g fiber; 1 g sugar; 418 mg phosphorous; 151 mg calcium; 2 mg iron; 311 mg sodium; 536 mg potassium; 797 IU vitamin A; 130 mg ATE vitamin E; 4 mg vitamin C; 113 mg cholesterol

Herbed Fish

185 CALORIES (26% FROM FAT, 69% FROM PROTEIN, 5% FROM CARB)

Here's a simple baked fish made flavorful by a combination of herbs and spices.

2 pounds (900 g) perch,
or other firm white fish

1 tablespoon (15 ml) olive oil

½ teaspoon garlic powder

½ teaspoon marjoram

⅓ teaspoon thyme

⅛ teaspoon white pepper

2 bay leaves

½ cup (80 g) chopped onion

½ cup (120 ml) white wine

—
Yield: 6 servings

Preheat oven to 350°F (180°C, gas mark 4). Wash fish, pat dry, and place in dish. Combine oil with and herbs and spices. Dribble over fish. Top with bay leaves and onion. Pour wine over all. Bake, uncovered, for 20 to 30 minutes or until fish flakes easily with a fork. Remove bay leaves before serving.

NUTRITIONAL ANALYSIS

EACH WITH: 148 g water; 28 g protein; 5 g total fat; 1 g saturated fat; 3 g monounsaturated fat; 1 g polyunsaturated fat; 2 g carb; 0 g fiber; 1 g sugar; 335 mg phosphorus; 169 mg calcium; 2 mg iron; 115 mg sodium; 450 mg potassium; 67 IU vitamin A; 2 mg vitamin C; 64 mg cholesterol

Oven-Poached Fish

486 CALORIES (19% FROM FAT, 74% FROM PROTEIN, 7% FROM CARB)

This is a really easy recipe that gives you fish that is a joy to eat, perfectly cooked, and subtly flavored.

4 halibut fillets,
1-inch (2½ cm) thick

¼ cup (16 g) fresh dill

4 slices lemon

2 tablespoons (10 g)
black peppercorns

¼ cup (60 ml) dry
white wine

Salt

—

Yield: 4 servings

Preheat oven to 450°F (230°C, or gas mark 8).. Place fish steaks in ungreased rectangular baking dish, 12 × 7 × 2 inches (30 × 18 × 5 cm). Sprinkle with salt. Place dill weed sprigs and lemon slice on each. Top with peppercorns. Pour wine over fish. Bake uncovered 20 to 25 minutes or until fish flakes easily.

NUTRITIONAL ANALYSIS

EACH WITH: 383 g water; 86 g Protein; 10 g total fat; 1 g saturated fat; 3 g monounsaturated fat; 3 g polyunsaturated fat; 8 g carb; 2 g fiber; 2 g sugar; 924 mg phosphorous; 223 mg calcium; 5 mg iron; 224 mg sodium; 1971 mg potassium; 706 IU vitamin A; 192 mg ATE vitamin E; 32 mg vitamin C; 131 mg cholesterol

Shrimp Kabobs

242 CALORIES (33% FROM FAT, 42% FROM PROTEIN, 26% FROM CARB)

These shrimp and veggies marinate in an unusual sauce containing mayonnaise and fresh cilantro. The resulting flavor is different, but it's different in a very good way.

⅓ cup (80 ml) Worcestershire sauce

½ cup (115 g) low-fat mayonnaise

½ cup (120 ml) lemon juice

2 cups (475 ml) clam juice

1 tablespoon (15 g) brown sugar

¼ cup (4 g) fresh chopped cilantro

1½ pounds (680 g) shrimp, peeled

1 cup (150 g) green bell pepper, cut in 1-inch (2½ cm) cubes

1 cup (150 g) red bell pepper, cut in 1-inch (2½ cm) cubes

1 onion, peeled and quartered

12 mushrooms

—
Yield: 6 servings

In oblong baking dish long enough to contain skewers, combine Worcestershire sauce, mayonnaise, lemon juice, clam juice, brown sugar, and cilantro, stirring briskly with fork to blend. On 6 long or 12 small skewers, arrange shrimp alternately with vegetables, ending with a mushroom to anchor (use 2 mushrooms if using long skewers, one at each end). Place skewers in pan with marinade, cover, and let stand 20 minutes or refrigerate overnight, turning often to coat all sides. Heat grill to medium. Remove kabobs from marinade and drain, reserving marinade. Cook kabobs over grill, about 4 minutes on each side, until seafood is cooked but still tender and vegetables are lightly browned. Heat remaining marinade to boiling in small saucepan and spoon over skewers before serving.

NUTRITIONAL ANALYSIS

EACH WITH: 226 g water; 25 g Protein; 9 g total fat; 1 g saturated fat; 0 g monounsaturated fat; 1 g polyunsaturated fat; 16 g carb; 2 g fiber; 7 g sugar; 313 mg phosphorous; 76 mg calcium; 4 mg iron; 465 mg sodium; 625 mg potassium; 1247 IU vitamin A; 61 mg ATE vitamin E; 91 mg vitamin C; 179 mg cholesterol

Shrimp Scampi

108 CALORIES (32% FROM FAT, 64% FROM PROTEIN, 4% FROM CARB)

Shrimp scampi is one of those dishes that seems to say "fancy", but it is really very easy to make. This recipe is ready to eat in only about 5 minutes.

1 teaspoon unsalted butter

2 teaspoons (10 ml) olive oil

3 garlic cloves, minced

1 pound (455 g) shrimp, peeled

¼ cup (60 ml) white wine

1 teaspoon lemon juice

¼ teaspoon ground black pepper

—
Yield: 6 servings

In sauté pan, melt butter and oil. Add garlic; sauté 1 minute. Add shrimp; sauté 1 minute. Add wine, lemon juice, and pepper. Sauté quickly until sauce reduces and shrimp turns pink, about 3 minutes. Do not overcook.

NUTRITIONAL ANALYSIS

EACH WITH: 67 g water; 15 g Protein; 3 g total fat; 1 g saturated fat; 1 g monounsaturated fat; 1 g polyunsaturated fat; 1 g carb; 0 g fiber; 0 g sugar; 157 mg phosphorous; 41 mg calcium; 2 mg iron; 113 mg sodium; 149 mg potassium; 156 IU vitamin A; 46 mg ATE vitamin E; 2 mg vitamin C; 117 mg cholesterol

Cioppino

272 CALORIES (35% FROM FAT, 52% FROM PROTEIN, 13% FROM CARB)

Cioppino is a traditional fisherman's stew made from a combination of whatever the catch was that day. Our version contains fish, shrimp, and clams, but feel free to add crab or other seafood or to use multiple varieties of fish.

1 pound (455 g) catfish

½ cup (75 g) green bell pepper, cut into ½-inch (1 cm) squares

2 tablespoons (20 g) onion, finely chopped

1 clove garlic, minced

1 tablespoon (15 ml) cooking oil

6 ounces (170 g) tomatoes, cut up

8 ounces (225 g) no-salt-added tomato sauce

½ cup (120 ml) dry white wine

3 tablespoons (12 g) fresh parsley

¼ teaspoon oregano, crushed

¼ teaspoon basil, crushed

Dash of pepper

12 ounces (340 g) shrimp, frozen or fresh

7 ounces (200 g) minced clams

—

Yield: 6 servings

Cut fillets into 1-inch (1 cm) pieces; set aside. In a 3 quart saucepan, cook green pepper, onion, and garlic in hot oil until onion is tender, not brown. Add undrained tomatoes, tomato sauce, wine, parsley, oregano, basil, and pepper. Bring to a boil. Reduce heat. Cover; simmer 20 minutes. Add fish pieces, shrimp, and undrained clams. Bring just to boiling. Reduce heat; cover and simmer 5 to 7 minutes or until fish and shrimp are done.

NUTRITIONAL ANALYSIS

EACH WITH: 215 g water; 33 g Protein; 10 g total fat; 2 g saturated fat; 4 g monounsaturated fat; 3 g polyunsaturated fat; 8 g carb; 1 g fiber; 2 g sugar; 408 mg phosphorous; 81 mg calcium; 12 mg iron; 170 mg sodium; 794 mg potassium; 846 IU vitamin A; 99 mg ATE vitamin E; 34 mg vitamin C; 144 mg cholesterol

Shrimp and Sausage Creole

349 CALORIES (72% FROM FAT, 20% FROM PROTEIN, 8% FROM CARB)

This dish of sausage and shrimp in a cream sauce gives a nice combination of creaminess with some heat. It has a flavor that is very like the Creole dishes served in some of New Orleans's most expensive restaurants.

1 tablespoon (15 ml) olive oil

10 shrimp

4 ounces (115 g) andouille sausage, sliced

1 cup (70 g) sliced mushrooms

½ cup (120 ml) skim milk

2 teaspoons (10 ml) Worcestershire sauce

1 teaspoon Creole seasoning

1 tablespoon (4 g) parsley

—

Yield: 2 servings

Heat olive oil in a heavy, large skillet over medium-high heat. Add shrimp and sausage and sauté until shrimp just turn pink, about 3 minutes. Using slotted spoon, transfer shrimp and sausage to a plate. Add mushrooms to same skillet and sauté until tender, about 4 minutes. Stir in milk, Worcestershire sauce, and seasoning. Simmer until sauce thickens, about 3 minutes. Return shrimp and sausage to skillet and simmer until shrimp are cooked through, about 1 minute. Sprinkle parsley over top. Serve over pasta.

NUTRITIONAL ANALYSIS

EACH WITH: 137 g water; 17 g protein; 28 g total fat; 8 g saturated fat; 15 g monounsaturated fat; 3 g polyunsaturated fat; 7 g carb; 0 g fiber; 1 g sugar; 108 mg calcium; 2 mg iron; 251 mg sodium; 429 mg potassium; 350 IU vitamin A; 14 mg vitamin C; 95 mg cholesterol

CHAPTER 7

Main Dishes:
Chicken and Turkey

---

*Most recent dietary recommendations include less red meat.
This chapter will make it easy to do. We have chicken
and turkey recipes from many different cultures. There should
be something here for everyone; probably a number of things.*

Rotisserie Chicken

71 CALORIES (18% FROM FAT, 30% FROM PROTEIN, 51% FROM CARB)

This recipe is equally good cooked in the oven or in a rotisserie if you have one.
Be forewarned that the honey will give you a very brown skin.

1 teaspoon paprika

1 teaspoon onion powder

½ teaspoon black pepper

½ teaspoon thyme

¼ teaspoon garlic powder

¼ cup (85 g) honey

1 large roasting chicken
(6 to 7 pounds or 2¾ to 3 kg)

—
Yield: 8 servings

Mix spices into honey. Brush onto chicken. Roast at 325°F (170°C, gas mark 3) until done, basting occasionally with pan juices.

NUTRITIONAL ANALYSIS

EACH WITH: 16 g water; 5 g protein; 1 g total fat; 0 g saturated fat; 1 g monounsaturated fat; 0 g polyunsaturated fat; 9 g carb; 0 g fiber; 9 g sugar; 7 mg calcium; 0 mg iron; 17 mg sodium; 67 mg potassium; 163 IU vitamin A; 0 mg vitamin C; 16 mg cholesterol

Cajun Beer Can Chicken

81 CALORIES (66% FROM FAT, 32% FROM PROTEIN, 2% FROM CARB)

This recipe has been around a while. This version adds a Cajun flavor. It makes a nice tender, juicy bird, either on the grill or in the oven. For a nonalcoholic chicken, substitute ginger ale or use nonalcoholic beer. You should use the indirect method, which means that you set up your fire so that it is hottest away from the food. On a charcoal grill, arrange it in two piles at opposite sides of the grill. Place a foil drip pan in the center of the grill between the mounds of embers. On a gas grill, if it has two burners, light one side on high and cook the chicken on the other.

1 chicken, 4 to 6 pounds
(1¾ to 2¾ kg)

3 tablespoons (12 g)
Cajun seasoning

12 ounces (355 ml) beer

3 cloves garlic

—
Yield: 8 servings

Remove and discard the fat from inside the body cavities of the chicken. Remove the package of giblets and set aside for another use. Rinse the chicken, inside and out, under cold running water; then drain and blot dry, inside and out, with paper towels. Sprinkle 1 tablespoon (4 g) of the seasoning inside the body and neck cavities; then rub the rest all over the skin of the bird. If you wish, rub another ½-tablespoon of the seasoning between the flesh and the skin. Cover and refrigerate the chicken while you preheat the grill. Pop the tab on the beer can. Using a "church key" type of can opener, punch six or seven holes in the top of the can. Pour out the top inch (2½ cm) of beer; drop the peeled garlic cloves into the holes in the can. Holding the chicken upright (wings at top, legs at bottom), with the opening of the body cavity down, insert the beer can into the lower cavity. Oil the grill grate. Stand the chicken up in the center of the hot grate, over the drip pan. Spread out the legs to form a sort of tripod to support the bird. Cover the grill and cook the chicken until fall-off-the-bone tender, about an hour, depending on size. Use a thermometer to check for doneness. The internal temperature should be 180°F (82°C). Using tongs, lift the bird to a cutting board or platter, holding a metal spatula underneath the beer can for support.

NUTRITIONAL ANALYSIS

EACH WITH: 25 g water; 6 g protein; 6 g total fat; 2 g saturated fat; 2 g monounsaturated fat; 1 g polyunsaturated fat; 0 g carb; 0 g fiber; 0 g sugar; 6 mg calcium; 0 mg iron; 25 mg sodium; 76 mg potassium; 48 IU vitamin A; 0 mg vitamin C; 27 mg cholesterol

Chicken Fingers

Easy-to-make baked chicken fingers are not only healthier than the typical fried ones, but they actually taste better according to many people.

213 CALORIES (47% FROM FAT, 46% FROM PROTEIN, 7% FROM CARB)

⅓ cup (10 g) cornflake crumbs

½ cup (55 g) pecans, finely chopped

1 tablespoon (1.3 g) parsley flakes

⅛ teaspoon garlic powder

12 ounces (340 g) boneless skinless chicken breast halves, cut into 1 × 3-inch (2½ × 7½ cm) strips

2 tablespoons (30 ml) skim milk

—

Yield: 5 servings

In a shallow dish, combine cornflake crumbs, pecans, parsley, and garlic powder. Dip chicken in milk and then roll in crumb mixture. Place in a 15 × 10 × 1-inch (38 × 25 × 2½ cm) baking pan. Bake in a 400°F (200°C, or gas mark 6). oven for 7 to 9 minutes or until chicken is tender and no longer pink.

NUTRITIONAL ANALYSIS

EACH WITH: 47 g water; 24 g protein; 11 g total fat; 2 g saturated fat; 6 g monounsaturated fat; 3 g polyunsaturated fat; 4 g carb; 1 g fiber; 1 g sugar; 207 mg phosphorous; 32 mg calcium; 1 mg iron; 59 mg sodium; 257 mg potassium; 67 IU vitamin A; 9 mg ATE vitamin E; 1 mg vitamin C; 62 mg cholesterol

Chicken Marsala

268 CALORIES (64% FROM FAT, 29% FROM PROTEIN, 7% FROM CARB)

This is a traditional Italian recipe, and it's one that is definitely worth trying.

4 boneless skinless
chicken breasts

4 tablespoons (55 g) butter,
divided

4 shallots, finely chopped

½ pound (225 g) mushrooms,
thinly sliced

¼ cup (60 ml) Marsala wine

½ cup (120 ml) heavy cream

1 teaspoon lemon juice

¼ teaspoon pepper

—
Yield: 4 servings

Using the flat (smooth) side of a meat mallet, pound the breasts to ¼ inch (½ cm) thickness. In a large frying pan, melt 2 teaspoons butter over medium heat. Add chicken and sauté, turning once, until lightly browned, about 2 minutes on each side. Remove and set aside. Melt remaining butter in pan. Add shallots and mushrooms. Cook until mushrooms are lightly browned, 3 to 5 minutes. Add Marsala and bring to a boil, scraping up any browned bits from bottom of pan. Add cream and lemon juice and return to a boil. Season with pepper to taste. Return chicken to pan and cook, turning in sauce, for about 3 minutes to reheat and finish cooking.

NUTRITIONAL ANALYSIS

EACH WITH: 128 g water; 19 g protein; 18 g total fat; 11 g saturated fat; 5 g monounsaturated fat; 1 g polyunsaturated fat; 5 g carb; 1 g fiber; 2 g sugar; 202 mg phosphorus; 25 mg calcium; 1 mg iron; 433 mg sodium; 393 mg potassium; 590 IU vitamin A; 3 mg vitamin C; 92 mg cholesterol

Chicken Piccata

159 CALORIES (49% FROM FAT, 47% FROM PROTEIN, 5% FROM CARB)

Here is another one of those classic recipes, updated to make it quicker and easier. Chicken is bathed in a lemon and vermouth sauce for an elegant flavor combination. Serve with rice or noodles.

4 boneless skinless chicken breasts

½ teaspoon black pepper, freshly ground

2 tablespoons (28 g) unsalted butter

1 teaspoon olive oil

½ cup (120 ml) low-sodium chicken broth

¼ cup (60 ml) vermouth

2 tablespoons (30 ml) fresh lemon juice

1 tablespoon (8.6 g) capers, drained, rinsed

—

Yield: 4 servings

Pat chicken dry. Season with pepper. Melt butter with oil in heavy large skillet over medium-high heat. Add chicken and cook until no longer pink, about 4 minutes per side. Remove from skillet; keep warm. Increase heat to high. Stir broth and vermouth into skillet. Boil until reduced by half, scraping up any browned bits. Remove from heat. Mix in lemon juice and capers. Place chicken on plates and pour sauce over. Garnish chicken with lemon slices, if desired.

NUTRITIONAL ANALYSIS

EACH WITH: 105 g water; 17 g Protein; 8 g total fat; 4 g saturated fat; 3 g monounsaturated fat; 1 g polyunsaturated fat; 2 g carb; 0 g fiber; 0 g sugar; 154 mg phosphorous; 15 mg calcium; 1 mg iron; 121 mg sodium; 233 mg potassium; 197 IU vitamin A; 52 mg ATE vitamin E; 5 mg vitamin C; 56 mg cholesterol

Slow Cooker Chicken in Tomato Cream Sauce

501 CALORIES (33% FROM FAT, 27% FROM PROTEIN, 40% FROM CARB)

This meal in a pot does take a little work near the end, but it is well worth it. Your family will love the creamy taste of the sauce with the chicken and pasta.

2 chicken breasts halves

2 tablespoons (30 ml) olive oil

¼ cup (25 g) green onions, chopped

1 teaspoon garlic, minced

14½ ounces (410 g) canned tomatoes, drained and chopped

1 tablespoon (4.5 g) basil

1 cup (235 ml) fat-free evaporated milk

2 egg yolks

¾ cup (75 g) parmesan cheese, grated

8 ounces (225 g) fettuccine

1 cup (130 g) frozen peas, thawed

1½ cup (105 g) mushrooms, sliced

—

Yield: 4 servings

In skillet, brown chicken breasts in olive oil. Place chicken in slow cooker. Add green onions, garlic, tomatoes, and basil. Cover and cook on Low 7 to 9 hours. Remove chicken and cut into pieces. Return chicken pieces to pot. Stir in cream, egg yolks, and Parmesan cheese. Cover and cook on high 30 minutes to thicken. While sauce is thickening, cook fettuccine according to package directions; drain. Add fettuccine, peas, and mushrooms. Cover and cook on high 30 to 60 minutes.

NUTRITIONAL ANALYSIS

EACH WITH: 267 g water; 34 g Protein; 18 g total fat; 6 g saturated fat; 8 g monounsaturated fat; 2 g polyunsaturated fat; 51 g carb; 4 g fiber; 13 g sugar; 533 mg phosphorous; 479 mg calcium; 5 mg iron; 719 mg sodium; 807 mg potassium; 1607 IU vitamin A; 151 mg ATE vitamin E; 17 mg vitamin C; 188 mg cholesterol

Quick Chicken and Mushroom Risotto

425 CALORIES (21% FROM FAT, 27% FROM PROTEIN, 52% FROM CARB)

Although not really risotto, which requires a specific preparation and particular kind of rice to get the traditional creaminess and texture, this recipe still give you that same sort of impression while taking less time and effort.

2 tablespoons (28 g) unsalted butter, divided

¾ pound (340 g) boneless skinless chicken breasts, cut in cubes

½ cup (80 g) onion, finely chopped

½ cup (65 g) carrot, sliced

1 cup (185 g) long grain rice, uncooked

14½ ounces (410 g) low-sodium chicken broth

1 can (10¾ ounces or 305 g) cream of mushroom soup

⅛ teaspoon pepper

½ cup (65 g) frozen peas

—

Yield: 4 servings

In 3-quart saucepan over medium-high heat, in 1 tablespoon (14 g) melted butter, cook chicken until browned, stirring often. Remove; set aside. In same saucepan, add remaining butter. Reduce heat to medium; cook onion, carrot, and rice until rice is browned, stirring constantly. Stir in broth, soup, and pepper. Heat to boiling. Reduce heat to low. Cover; cook 15 minutes, stirring occasionally. Add peas and reserved chicken. Cover; cook 5 minutes or until chicken is no longer pink, rice is tender, and liquid is absorbed, stirring occasionally.

NUTRITIONAL ANALYSIS

EACH WITH: 326 g water; 28 g Protein; 10 g total fat; 5 g saturated fat; 3 g monounsaturated fat; 1 g polyunsaturated fat; 55 g carb; 3 g fiber; 5 g sugar; 346 mg phosphorous; 59 mg calcium; 4 mg iron; 646 mg sodium; 944 mg potassium; 3318 IU vitamin A; 55 mg ATE vitamin E; 6 mg vitamin C; 68 mg cholesterol

Chicken Alfredo

133 CALORIES (21% FROM FAT, 49% FROM PROTEIN, 31% FROM CARB)

Kaye sent this recipe in. She comments that for the tomatoes, you could also use oven baked cherry tomatoes or sun-dried tomatoes.

2 boneless chicken breasts, cut in chunks

½ cup (90 g) chopped tomato

1 cup (70 g) sliced mushrooms

2 cloves garlic, minced

2 tablespoons (4 g) dried basil

1 slice low-sodium bacon, cooked and crumbled

8 ounces (225 g) no-salt-added tomato sauce

2 tablespoons (10 g) grated Parmesan cheese

4 ounces (120 ml) half-and-half

—
Yield: 4 servings

Sauté the chicken in olive oil until browned. Turn chicken and add tomato, mushrooms, and garlic and cook on medium heat until the mushrooms start to darken. Add basil, bacon, tomato sauce, and Parmesan. Heat on low for 15 minutes. Remove from heat. Add half-and-half to mixture. Mix well. Serve over pasta.

NUTRITIONAL ANALYSIS

EACH WITH: 135 g water; 13 g protein; 2 g total fat; 1 g saturated fat; 1 g monounsaturated fat; 0 g polyunsaturated fat; 8 g carb; 2 g fiber; 3 g sugar; 104 mg calcium; 1 mg iron; 107 mg sodium; 494 mg potassium; 572 IU vitamin A; 12 mg vitamin C; 36 mg cholesterol

Southwestern Skillet Supper

395 CALORIES (20% FROM FAT, 41% FROM PROTEIN, 39% FROM CARB)

This southwestern flavored chicken and bean dish is good served over rice and sprinkled with a little cheddar cheese.

1 pound (455 g) boneless skinless chicken breasts

2 tablespoons (30 ml) olive oil

1 cup (160 g) onion, chopped

2 teaspoons (5.2 g) chili powder

½ teaspoon cumin

½ teaspoon oregano

½ cup (120 ml) chicken broth

1½ cups (355 ml) low-sodium V8 juice

19 ounces (532 g) kidney beans

—

Yield: 4 servings

Cut the chicken into ½-inch (1 cm) pieces. In hot oil, cook chicken, onion, chili powder, cumin, and oregano until the chicken turns white. Stir in broth and juice. Heat until boiling and then reduce heat to low. Simmer 10 minutes. Add beans, liquid and all, stir, cover, and simmer for another 10 minutes. Stir occasionally.

NUTRITIONAL ANALYSIS

EACH WITH: 324 g water; 40 g Protein; 9 g total fat; 1 g saturated fat; 5 g monounsaturated fat; 1 g polyunsaturated fat; 39 g carb; 14 g fiber; 5 g sugar; 448 mg phosphorous; 130 mg calcium; 6 mg iron; 242 mg sodium; 1143 mg potassium; 1825 IU vitamin A; 7 mg ATE vitamin E; 32 mg vitamin C; 66 mg cholesterol

Cumin Crusted Chicken Salad

89 CALORIES (13% FROM FAT, 78% FROM PROTEIN, 8% FROM CARB)

I like the flavor of cumin, so this was a recipe that I just had to try. It turned out really well with the flavor on the chicken contrasting nicely with the vegetables.

¼ cup (45 g) tomato, chopped

3 tablespoons (25 g) cucumber, peeled and chopped

3 tablespoons (38 g) green pepper, chopped

1 tablespoon (10 g) red onion, chopped

1 small jalapeno pepper, chopped

1 tablespoon (6.6 g) cumin

1 teaspoon pepper

4 boneless skinless chicken breasts

1 tablespoon (15 ml) red wine vinegar

—

Yield: 4 servings

Combine tomato, cucumber, green pepper, red onion, and jalapeno pepper in a small bowl and set aside. Combine cumin and pepper. Rub all sides of chicken breasts with this. Place a large cast iron skillet over medium high heat until hot. Add chicken and cook 6 minutes on each side or until tender. Remove from skillet, reserving drippings in skillet. Set chicken aside. Add vinegar to pan drippings and cook 2 minutes, stirring constantly. Pour over reserved vegetable mixture, tossing well. Thinly slice each chicken breast diagonally across grain and arrange on individual serving plates. Serve with reserved vegetable mixture.

NUTRITIONAL ANALYSIS

EACH WITH: 80 g water; 17 g Protein; 1 g total fat; 0 g saturated fat; 0 g monounsaturated fat; 0 g polyunsaturated fat; 2 g carb; 0 g fiber; 1 g sugar; 153 mg phosphorous; 25 mg calcium; 2 mg iron; 50 mg sodium; 256 mg potassium; 167 IU vitamin A; 4 mg ATE vitamin E; 9 mg vitamin C; 41 mg cholesterol

Turkey Meat Loaf

191 CALORIES (23% FROM FAT, 49% FROM PROTEIN, 28% FROM CARB)

The glaze gives this a nice, sweet-tart taste without adding too many carbohydrates. The turkey is milder in flavor than beef, as well as being lower in fat.

1¼ pounds (570 g)
ground turkey

½ cup (60 g) low-sodium
bread crumbs

1 egg

1 tablespoon (4 g) parsley

½ teaspoon black pepper

½ teaspoon garlic powder

1 teaspoon onion powder

¼ cup (80 g) peach preserves

2 teaspoons Dijon mustard

—
Yield: 8 servings

Preheat oven to 350°F (180°C, gas mark 4). Combine first 8 ingredients in a large bowl and mix well. Shape mixture into a loaf on a baking sheet. Bake 45 minutes. Stir preserves and mustard together. Spread on top of loaf. Return to oven until internal temperature is 165°F (74°C), about 20 minutes.

NUTRITIONAL ANALYSIS

EACH WITH: 71 g water; 23 g protein; 5 g total fat; 1 g saturated fat; 1 g monounsaturated fat; 1 g polyunsaturated fat; 13 g carb; 1 g fiber; 6 g sugar; 42 mg calcium; 2 mg iron; 68 mg sodium; 293 mg potassium; 108 IU vitamin A; 4 mg vitamin C; 85 mg cholesterol

Noodles with Peanut Sauce and Chicken

403 CALORIES (39% FROM FAT, 37% FROM PROTEIN, 24% FROM CARB)

I used to be leery of Asian recipes that called for peanut butter. Then I tried this one and it was so good that I now actually consider finding a recipe with peanut butter a really good thing.

8 ounces (225 g) spaghetti

½ cup (130 g) peanut butter, creamy

2 tablespoons (30 ml) Reduced-Sodium Soy Sauce (see recipe in chapter 2)

1 teaspoon gingerroot, grated

½ cup (120 ml) low-sodium chicken broth

4 ounces (115 g) bean sprouts

1 cup (150 g) red bell peppers, sliced

2 green onion, sliced

1 pound (455 g) boneless skinless chicken breast

—
Yield: 4 servings

Cook spaghetti. Mix peanut butter, soy sauce, and gingerroot in saucepan. Add chicken broth. Add spaghetti, bean sprouts, bell pepper, and onion. Toss. Slice chicken into thin strips. Stir fry until no longer pink. Stir into spaghetti mixture.

NUTRITIONAL ANALYSIS

EACH WITH: 214 g water; 38 g protein; 18 g total fat; 3 g saturated fat; 8 g monounsaturated fat; 5 g polyunsaturated fat; 25 g carb; 6 g fiber; 5 g sugar; 404 mg phosphorous; 43 mg calcium; 2 mg iron; 131 mg sodium; 669 mg potassium; 1194 IU vitamin A; 7 mg ATE vitamin E; 49 mg vitamin C; 66 mg cholesterol

Chicken Mole

343 CALORIES (31% FROM FAT, 37% FROM PROTEIN, 32% FROM CARB)

Chicken mole can be a long involved recipe. We shortened the time but kept the traditional flavor by using the microwave to prepare the sauce and cook the chicken.

2 teaspoons (4 g) cocoa powder, unsweetened

1½ teaspoon chili powder

½ teaspoon cumin, ground

½ teaspoon oregano, dried crushed

8 ounces (225 g) no-salt-added tomato sauce

¼ cup (40 g) onion, finely chopped

3 cloves garlic, minced

1 pound (455 g) boneless skinless chicken breast, cut into bite-sized pieces

4 ounces (115 g) green chili peppers, diced, drained

2 tablespoons (14 g) almonds, toasted sliced

4 flour tortillas

½ cup (90 g) tomato, chopped

½ cup (28 g) lettuce, shredded

1 avocado, sliced

—
Yield: 4 servings

In a 1½ quart (1.5 L) microwave-safe casserole, combine cocoa powder, chili powder, cumin, oregano, and salt. Stir in tomato sauce, onion and garlic. Micro-cook, covered, on 100% power (high) for 2 to 3 minutes or until mixture is bubbly around edges, stirring once. Stir in chicken and chili peppers. Cover; cook on high for 8 to 10 minutes (10 to 12 minutes for low-wattage ovens) or until chicken is tender and no longer pink inside, stirring every 3 minutes. Garnish with almonds. To serve: warm tortillas, fill with chicken mixture, tomato, lettuce, and avocado.

EACH WITH: 231 g water; 32 g Protein; 12 g total fat; 2 g saturated fat; 6 g monounsaturated fat; 2 g polyunsaturated fat; 28 g carb; 6 g fiber; 4 g sugar; 341 mg phosphorous; 97 mg calcium; 4 mg iron; 400 mg sodium; 891 mg potassium; 797 IU vitamin A; 7 mg ATE vitamin E; 26 mg vitamin C; 66 mg cholesterol

Chicken Fried Rice

360 CALORIES (44% FROM FAT, 30% FROM PROTEIN, 26% FROM CARB)

This is our favorite recipe for fried rice. It's a little more work than some recipes, but I think the result is worth it.

1 pound (455 g) boneless skinless chicken breast

½ teaspoon cornstarch

1 dash white pepper

1 cup (50 g) bean sprouts

5 tablespoons (75 ml) vegetable oil

2 eggs, slightly beaten

2½ ounces (70 g) sliced mushrooms

3 cups (495 g) white rice

2 tablespoons (30 ml) Reduced-Sodium Soy Sauce (see recipe in chapter 2)

2 green onions with tops, sliced

—

Yield: 5 servings

Cut chicken into ¼-inch (5 mm) pieces. Toss together chicken, cornstarch, and dash white pepper. Heat wok until very hot. Add 1 tablespoon (15 ml) oil and coat sides. Add eggs. Cook and stir until eggs are thickened throughout but still moist. Remove eggs from wok. Wash and dry wok thoroughly. Reheat wok, add 2 tablespoons (30 ml) oil, and coat sides. Add chicken and stir-fry until chicken turns white. Add bean sprouts and mushrooms. Stir-fry 1 minute. Remove from wok and drain. Heat wok very hot, add 2 tablespoons oil, and coat sides. Add rice and stir-fry 1 minute. Stir in soy sauce. Add eggs, chicken mixture, and green onions and stir-fry 30 seconds.

NUTRITIONAL ANALYSIS

EACH WITH: 202 g water; 27 g Protein; 17 g total fat; 3 g saturated fat; 5 g monounsaturated fat; 8 g polyunsaturated fat; 23 g carb; 1 g fiber; 1 g sugar; 249 mg phosphorous; 28 mg calcium; 1 mg iron; 131 mg sodium; 324 mg potassium; 130 IU vitamin A; 37 mg ATE vitamin E; 1 mg vitamin C; 147 mg cholesterol

Turkey Sausage and Pepper Patties

284 CALORIES (34% FROM FAT, 61% FROM PROTEIN, 4% FROM CARB)

I happen to be one of the people who think that ground turkey tends to be pretty plain and lacking in real flavor. So I came up with this combination, which quite nicely solves the problem for me.

1 tablespoon (15 ml) olive oil

½ cup (75 g) green pepper, finely minced

½ cup (80 g) onion, finely minced

1¼ pounds (570 g) ground turkey

¼ teaspoon sage

¼ teaspoon thyme

¼ teaspoon marjoram

¼ teaspoon pepper

½ teaspoon fennel seeds

—
Yield: 4 servings

Heat oil in skillet; add peppers and onions and cook until tender, about 10 minutes. Cool. Combine peppers and onions with turkey and remaining ingredients, mixing well. Chill an hour or so to blend flavors. Form into 4 patties. Cook in nonstick skillet until lightly browned on both sides.

NUTRITIONAL ANALYSIS

EACH WITH: 127 g water; 42 g Protein; 11 g total fat; 3 g saturated fat; 4 g monounsaturated fat; 2 g polyunsaturated fat; 3 g carb; 1 g fiber; 1 g sugar; 313 mg phosphorous; 47 mg calcium; 3 mg iron; 101 mg sodium; 490 mg potassium; 83 IU vitamin A; 0 mg ATE vitamin E; 17 mg vitamin C; 108 mg cholesterol

CHAPTER 8

Main Dishes: Beef, Pork, and Lamb

Despite what I said in the chicken chapter about eating less red meat, we still eat it on a regular basis. But that doesn't mean it needs to be unhealthy. This chapter contains recipes that not only taste great but are low in GI and saturated fat. We have recipes for the grill, meat loaves and meatballs, and stews.

Beef Burgundy

476 CALORIES (43% FROM FAT, 35% FROM PROTEIN, 22% FROM CARB)

This is a great beef and noodles dish, and it's so easy to prepare in your slow cooker. The beef gets very tender from the long cooking process.

4 slices low-sodium bacon

2 pounds (900 g) beef stew meat

1 cup (130 g) carrots, cut into chunks

1 onion, sliced

½ cup (64 g) all-purpose flour

½ teaspoon marjoram

¼ teaspoon garlic powder

¼ teaspoon black pepper

1 cup (235 ml) low-sodium beef broth

½ cup (120 ml) burgundy wine

1 tablespoon (15 ml) Worcestershire sauce

3 cups (210 g) sliced mushrooms

8 ounces (225 g) uncooked egg noodles

2 tablespoons (8 g) fresh parsley (optional)

—

Yield: 8 servings

Cook bacon until crisp; drain and crumble. Place beef, bacon, carrots, and onions in the bottom of the slow cooker. Whisk together flour, marjoram, garlic powder, and pepper with broth, wine, and Worcestershire sauce. Pour mixture into slow cooker. Cook on high for 1 hour. Reduce to low and cook for 5 to 6 hours. Add mushrooms to slow cooker. Cook on high for 30 minutes or until mushrooms are tender. While mushrooms are cooking, prepare noodles according to package directions. Serve beef over noodles and garnished with parsley, if desired.

NUTRITIONAL ANALYSIS

EACH WITH: 195 g water; 40 g protein; 22 g total fat; 8 g saturated fat; 9 g monounsaturated fat; 1 g polyunsaturated fat; 15 g carb; 1 g fiber; 2 g sugar; 32 mg calcium; 5 mg iron; 140 mg sodium; 563 mg potassium; 2,023 IU vitamin A; 7 mg vitamin C; 137 mg cholesterol

Sweet and Sour Meatballs

402 CALORIES (53% FROM FAT, 25% FROM PROTEIN, 22% FROM CARB)

These tasty meatballs have a fairly traditional sweet and sour flavor and are great served over rice.

1½ pounds (680 g) lean ground beef

⅔ cup (86 g) cracker crumbs

⅓ cup (60 g) onion, minced

1 egg

¼ teaspoon ginger

¼ cup (60 ml) milk

1 tablespoon (15 ml) olive oil

2 tablespoons (16 g) cornstarch

13 ounces (365 g) pineapple tidbits, drained (reserve syrup)

½ cup (8 g) brown sugar substitute, such as Splenda

⅓ cup (80 ml) cider vinegar

⅓ cup (50 g) green bell pepper, chopped

—
Yield: 6 servings

Mix thoroughly beef, crumbs, onion, egg, ginger, and milk. Shape mixture by rounded teaspoonfuls into balls. Heat oil in large skillet; brown and cook meatballs. Remove meatballs; keep warm. Pour fat from skillet. Mix cornstarch and sugar. Stir in reserved pineapple syrup and vinegar. Pour into skillet; cook over medium heat, stirring constantly until mixture thickens and boils. Add meatballs, pineapple tidbits, and bell pepper; heat through.

NUTRITIONAL ANALYSIS

EACH WITH: 172 g water; 25 g Protein; 24 g total fat; 9 g saturated fat; 11 g monounsaturated fat; 2 g polyunsaturated fat; 22 g carb; 1 g fiber; 10 g sugar; 214 mg phosphorous; 60 mg calcium; 3 mg iron; 97 mg sodium; 489 mg potassium; 131 IU vitamin A; 21 mg ATE vitamin E; 12 mg vitamin C; 113 mg cholesterol

Braised Short Ribs

596 CALORIES (49% FROM FAT, 42% FROM PROTEIN, 9% FROM CARB)

Beef short ribs are browned and then given a long, slow braising in the slow cooker, resulting in falling off the bone tenderness.

4 pounds (1.8 kg) beef short ribs

½ cup (63 g) flour

1½ teaspoons paprika

½ teaspoon dry mustard

1½ cups (240 g) onion, sliced and separated into rings

1 clove garlic, chopped

1 cup (235 ml) beer or beef broth

—

Yield: 6 servings

Place short ribs in skillet and brown to remove fat; drain well. Combine flour with the paprika and dry mustard; toss with short ribs. Place in slow cooker. Place remaining ingredients over beef. Cook on low for 8 to 10 hours.

NUTRITIONAL ANALYSIS

EACH WITH: 283 g water; 59 g Protein; 31 g total fat; 13 g saturated fat; 13 g monounsaturated fat; 1 g polyunsaturated fat; 13 g carb; 1 g fiber; 2 g sugar; 605 mg phosphorous; 38 mg calcium; 7 mg iron; 200 mg sodium; 1174 mg potassium; 304 IU vitamin A; 0 mg ATE vitamin E; 3 mg vitamin C; 178 mg cholesterol

Home-Style Meat Loaf

363 CALORIES (51% FROM FAT, 28% FROM PROTEIN, 21% FROM CARB)

An iron-rich food like meat loaf can help keep you warm on winter nights. When researchers at the U.S. Department of Agriculture deprived a group of women of iron, they became chilled more quickly when exposed to lower temperatures. Besides, it tastes good.

¾ cup (180 g) ketchup, divided

½ cup (40 g) quick-cooking oats

¼ cup (40 g) minced onion

2 tablespoons (8 g) chopped parsley

1 tablespoon (15 g) brown sugar

¼ teaspoon black pepper

2 large egg whites, lightly beaten

1½ pounds (680 g) ground round

—

Yield: 6 servings

Preheat oven to 350°F (180°C, gas mark 4). Combine ½ cup (120 g) ketchup, oats, and next 6 ingredients (oats through egg whites) in a large bowl. Add meat; stir just until blended. Shape meat mixture into an 8 × 4-inch (20 × 10 cm) loaf on a broiler pan coated with nonstick vegetable oil spray. Brush remaining ketchup over meat loaf. Bake 1½ hours or until done.

NUTRITIONAL ANALYSIS

EACH WITH: 110 g water; 25 g protein; 20 g total fat; 8 g saturated fat; 9 g monounsaturated fat; 1 g polyunsaturated fat; 19 g carb; 2 g fiber; 9 g sugar; 243 mg phosphorus; 27 mg calcium; 3 mg iron; 528 mg sodium; 536 mg potassium; 386 IU vitamin A; 7 mg vitamin C; 78 mg cholesterol

Easy Cheeseburger Pie

261 CALORIES (50% FROM FAT, 29% FROM PROTEIN, 21% FROM CARB)

This is a variation of the Bisquick impossible pie recipe with most of the sodium removed. The nice part about this is you can quickly mix it up and put it in the oven without worrying about making pie crust.

1 pound (455 g) lean ground beef

1 onion, chopped

¼ teaspoon black pepper

½ cup (64 g) flour

¾ teaspoon sodium-free baking powder

2 tablespoons (28 g) unsalted butter

1 cup (235 ml) skim milk

1 egg

1 tomato, sliced

4 ounces (115 g) Swiss cheese, shredded

—
Yield: 6 servings

Cook beef and onion until beef is brown and onion soft. Stir in pepper. Place in bottom of a greased 9-inch (23 cm) pie plate. Stir together dry ingredients. Cut in butter. Stir in milk and egg. Pour over beef mixture. Bake at 400°F (200°C, gas mark 6) for 25 minutes. Top with tomato slices and cheese. Cook an additional 5 to 8 minutes until cheese melts and knife inserted in center comes out clean.

NUTRITIONAL ANALYSIS

EACH WITH: 120 g water; 19 g protein; 14 g total fat; 6 g saturated fat; 5 g monounsaturated fat; 1 g polyunsaturated fat; 14 g carb; 1 g fiber; 2 g sugar; 105 mg calcium; 2 mg iron; 81 mg sodium; 429 mg potassium; 456 IU vitamin A; 5 mg vitamin C; 98 mg cholesterol

Braised Sirloin Tips

542 CALORIES (45% FROM FAT, 53% FROM PROTEIN, 3% FROM CARB)

These tips are very tender and flavorful.

2 pounds (900 g) sirloin tips

1 tablespoon (15 ml) olive oil

⅓ cup (80 ml) cranberry juice

1 can (10½ ounces or 295 g) beef consommé

3 tablespoons (45 ml) Reduced-Sodium Soy Sauce (see chapter 2)

⅛ teaspoon garlic powder

⅛ teaspoon ginger

Cornstarch

—
Yield: 4 servings

Cut sirloin tips into bite-size pieces; brown on all sides in oil in skillet; add juice, consommé, soy sauce, garlic, and ginger. Simmer for 1½ hours or until tender. Blend small amount of cornstarch with water (use cold so it won't lump). Stir into beef until thickened, stirring constantly.

NUTRITIONAL ANALYSIS

EACH WITH: 234 g water; 69 g protein; 26 g total fat; 9 g saturated fat; 10 g monounsaturated fat; 3 g polyunsaturated fat; 4 g carb; 0 g fiber; 0 g sugar; 535 mg phosphorus; 53 mg calcium; 5 mg iron; 1386 mg sodium; 865 mg potassium; 2 IU vitamin A; 2 mg vitamin C; 166 mg cholesterol

Bulgogi

374 CALORIES (45% FROM FAT, 48% FROM PROTEIN, 6% FROM CARB)

I spent some time in Korea when I was in the Army. My favorite Korean food was bulgogi, beef skewers marinated in a spicy ginger, red pepper, and soy-based sauce. At that time, Korean food wasn't well known in the United States, but now there are a number of Korean restaurants serving bulgogi and other dishes. You can also make a good bulgogi at home, and if your family is like mine, they'll be glad you did.

2 pound (900 g) flank steak

1½ tablespoons (12 g) gingerroot, grated

2 tablespoons (30 ml) olive oil

1 teaspoon sesame oil

2 teaspoons (5.4 g) sesame seeds

⅔ cups Reduced-Sodium Teriyaki Sauce (see chapter 2)

2 garlic cloves, minced

½ teaspoon red pepper flakes

—
Yield: 6 servings

Lightly freeze steak and slice into thin slices. Mix all but sesame seeds together and marinate meat at least 3 hours. Skewer and broil or barbecue. Sprinkle with sesame seeds.

NUTRITIONAL ANALYSIS

EACH WITH: 120 g water; 44 g Protein; 18 g total fat; 6 g saturated fat; 9 g monounsaturated fat; 2 g polyunsaturated fat; 6 g carb; 0 g fiber; 4 g sugar; 376 mg phosphorous; 41 mg calcium; 4 mg iron; 97 mg sodium; 597 mg potassium; 61 IU vitamin A; 0 mg ATE vitamin E; 0 mg vitamin C; 83 mg cholesterol

Memphis Spareribs

529 CALORIES (45% FROM FAT, 15% FROM PROTEIN, 39% FROM CARB)

These ribs are done in the traditional way, cooked most of the way with just a spice rub and then "mopped" with sauce near the end. This helps to keep the meat from getting too dried out. I personally prefer to smoke the ribs until they are nearly done and then move them to the grill for the last 20 minutes or so to sear the sauce into them.

2 pounds (900 g) pork spareribs

¼ cup (60 ml) cider vinegar

RUB

½ cup (115 g) brown sugar

1½ teaspoons black pepper

1 teaspoon cayenne pepper

SAUCE

8 ounces (225 g) no-salt-added tomato sauce

½ cup (120 ml) cider vinegar

¼ cup (85 g) honey

1 teaspoon onion powder

1 teaspoon dry mustard

1 teaspoon garlic powder

½ teaspoon cayenne pepper

—
Yield: 4 servings

Brush ribs with vinegar. Mix rub ingredients together and rub into ribs. Smoke or grill until done. While ribs are cooking, combine sauce ingredients. Brush with sauce during the last 30 minutes of cooking.

NUTRITIONAL ANALYSIS

EACH WITH: 162 g water; 21 g protein; 27 g total fat; 10 g saturated fat; 12 g monounsaturated fat; 3 g polyunsaturated fat; 53 g carb; 1 g fiber; 49 g sugar; 78 mg calcium; 3 mg iron; 106 mg sodium; 694 mg potassium; 487 IU vitamin A; 8 mg vitamin C; 88 mg cholesterol

Zucchini Stuffed Pork Chops

187 CALORIES (36% FROM FAT, 57% FROM PROTEIN, 7% FROM CARB)

Boneless pork chops are stuffed with a flavorful vegetable mixture, giving maximum flavor and a very low GI.

1½ cup (188 g) zucchini, shredded

1 clove garlic, crushed

2 tablespoons (10 g) parmesan cheese, grated

¼ teaspoon black pepper

4 boneless pork loin chops

1 teaspoon (5 ml) olive oil

½ cup (120 ml) dry white wine or chicken broth

1 tablespoon (11 g) Dijon mustard

—
Yield: 4 servings

Squeeze zucchini with paper towels to remove moisture. Spray 10-inch (25 cm) nonstick skillet with nonstick cooking spray. Cook zucchini and garlic in skillet over medium heat about 3 minutes or until tender. Stir in cheese and pepper. Remove zucchini mixture from skillet; cool. Trim fat from pork chops. Flatten each pork chop to ¼-inch (5 mm) thickness between waxed paper or plastic wrap. Spread one-fourth of the zucchini mixture over each piece of pork. Roll up; secure with wooden picks. Add oil and pork rolls to skillet. Cover and cook over medium heat 15 to 20 minutes, turning once, until done. Remove wooden picks. Remove pork rolls from skillet; keep warm. Add wine to skillet. Cook over high heat 2 to 3 minutes or until reduced by half. Stir in mustard. Pour sauce over pork rolls.

NUTRITIONAL ANALYSIS

EACH WITH: 148 g water; 23 g Protein; 7 g total fat; 2 g saturated fat; 3 g monounsaturated fat; 1 g polyunsaturated fat; 3 g carb; 1 g fiber; 1 g sugar; 270 mg phosphorous; 60 mg calcium; 1 g iron; 148 mg sodium; 527 mg potassium; 117 IU vitamin A; 6 mg ATE vitamin E; 9 mg vitamin C; 66 mg cholesterol

Schnitzel

372 CALORIES (54% FROM FAT, 29% FROM PROTEIN, 17% FROM CARB)

This is properly called Wiener Schnitzel if you use veal chops and Schweineschnitzel if you use pork, which I do. Some people serve this with a fried egg placed on top of the schnitzel.

2 tablespoons (30 ml) olive oil

4 pork loin chops, boneless

2 eggs

½ cup (60 g) low-sodium fine bread crumbs

¼ teaspoon pepper

2 lemons

—

Yield: 4 servings

Heat the oil in a large skillet at medium-high heat. Place each chop between 2 sheets of plastic and pound with the smooth side of a meat tenderizer until thin (¼ inch to ½ inch or ½ to 1 cm thick). Beat the 2 eggs in a bowl that is wide enough to dip the meat into. Spread the bread crumbs onto a plate or flat surface. Take each cutlet, season with pepper, and dip both sides of meat into eggs to coat. Then coat the entire cutlet with the bread crumbs. Place in hot oil and cook on both sides until golden brown. It only takes about 1 to 2 minutes per side. Serve each cutlet with half a lemon on the side. Some people go ahead and squeeze the lemon onto the schnitzel before serving.

NUTRITIONAL ANALYSIS

EACH WITH: 112 g water; 28 g protein; 23 g total fat; 7 g saturated fat; 12 g monounsaturated fat; 2 g polyunsaturated fat; 16 g carb; 3 g fiber; 1 g sugar; 274 mg phosphorus; 96 mg calcium; 2 mg iron; 109 mg sodium; 465 mg potassium; 159 IU vitamin A; 42 mg vitamin C; 184 mg cholesterol

Pork Turnovers

158 CALORIES (57% FROM FAT, 19% FROM PROTEIN, 23% FROM CARB)

The preparation of these turnovers is similar to many Latin American meat turnovers, but the flavor is American, with mustard providing a little zip. If you like them spicier, add a small amount of red pepper flakes to the meat mixture.

8 teaspoons (112 g) unsalted butter

¾ cup (94 g) flour

3 tablespoons (45 ml) water

4 ounces (120 g) ground pork, cooked and crumbled

2 ounces (60 g) Monterey jack cheese shredded

1 teaspoon prepared mustard

1 egg, separated

1 tablespoon (15 ml) skim milk

—
Yield: 8 servings

In small bowl, with pastry blender or 2 knives, cut margarine into flour until mixture resembles cornmeal; sprinkle with ice water and use fork to mix until it forms soft dough. Roll dough between 2 sheets of wax paper to form a rectangle about ¼ inch (5 mm) thick; remove paper and use 2-inch (5 cm) diameter cookie cutter to cut dough into rounds. Roll scraps of dough and continue cutting until all dough has been used (should yield 24 rounds). Combine pork, cheese, and mustard in small bowl and set aside. Preheat oven to 375°F (190°C, or gas mark 5). Beat egg white lightly and brush an equal amount onto each pastry round. Spoon an equal amount of the meat mixture (about ½ rounded teaspoon) onto center of each round; fold pastry over, turnover-fashion, to enclose filling. Press edges of dough together to seal. Transfer turnovers to nonstick cookie sheet. Add milk to egg yolk and beat lightly; brush an equal amount of mixture over each turnover. Bake until turnovers are golden brown, 15 to 20 minutes.

NUTRITIONAL ANALYSIS

EACH WITH: 24 g water; 8 g Protein; 10 g total fat; 5 g saturated fat; 3 g monounsaturated fat; 1 g polyunsaturated fat; 9 g carb; 0 g fiber; 0 g sugar; 91 mg phosphorous; 66 mg calcium; 1 mg iron; 62 mg sodium; 84 mg potassium; 220 IU vitamin A; 58 mg ATE vitamin E; 0 mg vitamin C; 56 mg cholesterol

Stuffed Acorn Squash

410 CALORIES (40% FROM FAT, 24% FROM PROTEIN, 36% FROM CARB)

This acorn squash stuffed with a ground pork mixture is a favorite around our house. For variety you can also use ground turkey.

1 acorn squash, about 1 pound (455 g)

¼ cup (25 g) celery, chopped

¼ teaspoon cinnamon

1 slice whole wheat bread, cubed

6 ounces (170 g) ground pork

¼ cup (40 g) chopped onion

¼ teaspoon curry powder

½ cup (125 g) applesauce, unsweetened

—
Yield: 2 servings

Spray a 10 × 6 × 2-inch (25 × 15 × 5 cm) baking dish with nonstick cooking spray. Halve squash; discard seeds. Place squash, cut side down, in baking dish. Bake, uncovered, in 350°F (180°C, or gas mark 4) oven 50 minutes. While that is roasting, prepare the stuffing. In a skillet, cook pork, celery, and onion until meat is no longer pink and vegetables are tender. Drain fat. Stir in curry powder and cinnamon; cook 1 minute more. Stir in applesauce and bread cubes. Turn squash cut side up in dish. Place stuffing in squash halves. Bake uncovered, 20 minutes more.

NUTRITIONAL ANALYSIS

EACH WITH: 322 g water; 25 g Protein; 18 g total fat; 7 g saturated fat; 8 g monounsaturated fat; 2 g polyunsaturated fat; 38 g carb; 5 g fiber; 8 g sugar; 303 mg phosphorous; 124 mg calcium; 3 mg iron; 146 mg sodium; 1192 mg potassium; 875 IU vitamin A; 2 mg ATE vitamin E; 27 mg vitamin C; 80 mg cholesterol

Lamb Stew

534 CALORIES (35% FROM FAT, 51% FROM PROTEIN, 14% FROM CARB)

We don't eat lamb very often, but this stew is one recipe that has proved popular when lamb is on sale.

1 tablespoon (15 ml) olive oil

2 cups (320 g) onion, thinly sliced

1 tablespoon (10 g) garlic, minced

¼ cup (60 ml) red wine vinegar

2 pounds (900 g) lamb shoulder, trimmed and cut into 1-inch (2½ cm) cubes

14 ounces (400 g) no-salt-added tomatoes

2 tablespoons (32 g) no-salt-added tomato paste

1 teaspoon basil

1 teaspoon oregano

2 bay leaves

¼ teaspoon black pepper

1 cup (150 g) red bell pepper, sliced

1 cup (150 g) green bell pepper, sliced

⅓ cup (20 g) fresh parsley, finely minced

—
Yield: 4 servings

In Dutch oven, heat oil. Sauté onions and garlic until onions are soft, about 2 minutes. Stir in vinegar and cook for 1 to 2 minutes over medium heat, scraping any browned bits from the bottom. Add lamb, tomatoes, tomato paste, basil, oregano, bay leaves, salt and pepper to taste. Stir well to blend. Bring to boil, reduce heat, cover, and cook until lamb is fork tender, about 1 to 1½ hours. Remove bay leaves; stir in the red and green peppers. Cover and simmer over medium heat until peppers are crisp-tender, another 5 to 8 minutes. Remove the bay leaves and stir in the parsley just before serving.

NUTRITIONAL ANALYSIS

EACH WITH: 404 g water; 67 g Protein; 21 g total fat; 7 g saturated fat; 9 g monounsaturated fat; 2 g polyunsaturated fat; 18 g carb; 5 g fiber; 9 g sugar; 583 mg phosphorous; 108 mg calcium; 8 mg iron; 204 mg sodium; 1344 mg potassium; 2002 IU vitamin A; 0 mg ATE vitamin E; 102 mg vitamin C; 204 mg cholesterol

Glazed Pork Roast

173 CALORIES (22% FROM FAT, 57% FROM PROTEIN, 21% FROM CARB)

I actually grill this when it's warm enough. If you want to do that, it's best to grill with indirect heat. Place a pan of water under the roast and mound the charcoal around it. Close the grill to hold in the heat and smoke. This makes excellent sandwiches when it's cold and sliced thinly.

2 pounds (900 g) pork tenderloin

¼ cup (85 g) honey

1 tablespoon (9 g) dry mustard

¼ cup (60 ml) white wine vinegar

1 teaspoon chili powder

—

Yield: 8 servings

Mix together last 4 ingredients. Trim excess fat from pork roast. Brush with glaze. Roast at 350°F (180°C, gas mark 4) until done, 1 to 1½ hours, occasionally brushing with remaining glaze.

NUTRITIONAL ANALYSIS

EACH WITH: 94 g water; 24 g protein; 4 g total fat; 1 g saturated fat; 2 g monounsaturated fat; 0 g polyunsaturated fat; 9 g carb; 0 g fiber; 9 g sugar; 258 mg phosphorus; 9 mg calcium; 2 mg iron; 61 mg sodium; 436 mg potassium; 101 IU vitamin A; 1 mg vitamin C; 74 mg cholesterol

CHAPTER 9

Salads and Salad Dressings

Salads fit perfectly into our low-GI lifestyle with their emphasis on vegetables and their typically low carbohydrate contents. This chapter includes a selection of both side-dish salads and main-dish salad meals. We try to have at least one salad meal a week during the summer when fresh vegetables are plentiful and we don't feel like cooking. There also are a couple of salad dressing recipes. Most commercial salad dressing is not that bad nutritionally, but these are some we like that are a little different from the ones in the grocery store.

Buttermilk Dill Dressing

79 CALORIES (84% FROM FAT, 5% FROM PROTEIN, 11% FROM CARB)

This is a good dressing when you are having fish or chicken.

¼ cup (60 g) low-sodium mayonnaise

½ cup (120 ml) buttermilk

1 tablespoon (10 g) minced onion

2 teaspoons (2 g) dill

1 teaspoon basil

1 tablespoon (4 g) parsley

¼ teaspoon garlic powder

Dash cayenne pepper

—

Yield: 6 servings

Combine ingredients in a blender or food processor and process until smooth. Refrigerate several hours or overnight before serving to allow flavor to develop.

NUTRITIONAL ANALYSIS

EACH WITH: 21 g water; 1 g protein; 7 g total fat; 1 g saturated fat; 2 g monounsaturated fat; 3 g polyunsaturated fat; 2 g carb; 0 g fiber; 1 g sugar; 37 mg calcium; 0 mg iron; 25 mg sodium; 68 mg potassium; 115 IU vitamin A; 2 mg vitamin C; 6 mg cholesterol

TIP

Replace one teaspoon of the dill with oregano or Italian seasoning for a good ranch-type dressing.

Sun-Dried Tomato Vinaigrette

70 CALORIES (91% FROM FAT, 1% FROM PROTEIN, 8% FROM CARB)

This dressing has a nice flavor, but it also contains a fair amount of fat, which I've not made any attempt to reduce.

3 tablespoons (45 ml) white wine vinegar

¼ cup (14 g) chopped sun-dried tomatoes

1 teaspoon Worcestershire sauce

1 clove garlic, minced

½ teaspoon sugar

¼ tablespoon white pepper

⅓ cup (80 ml) olive oil

—
Yield: 8 servings

Shake ingredients together in a jar with a tight-fitting lid.

NUTRITIONAL ANALYSIS

EACH WITH: 7 g water; 0 g protein; 7 g total fat; 1 g saturated fat; 5 g monounsaturated fat; 1 g polyunsaturated fat; 1 g carb; 0 g fiber; 0 g sugar; 6 mg phosphorus; 3 mg calcium; 0 mg iron; 16 mg sodium; 63 mg potassium; 45 IU vitamin A; 5 mg vitamin C; 0 mg cholesterol

Balsamic Vinaigrette

42 CALORIES (96% FROM FAT, 1% FROM PROTEIN, 3% FROM CARB)

This dressing has a more distinct flavor than many of the balsamic dressing sold commercially. The mustard seems to raise it to a higher level.

1 tablespoon (11 g) Dijon mustard

¼ cup (60 ml) balsamic vinegar

2 tablespoons (30 ml) water

2 tablespoons (30 ml) fresh lemon juice

¼ teaspoon pepper

¼ teaspoon dried tarragon

1 clove garlic, minced

¼ cup (60 ml) olive oil

—

Yield: 12 servings

In a jar, combine the mustard, vinegar, water, lemon juice, pepper, tarragon, and garlic. Shake well to combine. Add oils and shake again. Chill before serving.

NUTRITIONAL ANALYSIS

EACH WITH: 11 g water; 0 g Protein; 5 g total fat; 1 g saturated fat; 3 g monounsaturated fat; 0 g polyunsaturated fat; 0 g carb; 0 g fiber; 0 g sugar; 2 mg phosphorous; 2 mg calcium; 0 mg iron; 15 mg sodium; 9 mg potassium; 4 IU vitamin A; 0 mg ATE vitamin E; 1 mg vitamin C; 0 mg cholesterol

Poppy Seed Dressing

158 CALORIES (94% FROM FAT, 1% FROM PROTEIN, 5% FROM CARB)

This dressing is good on just about any kind of salad, but it seems to be particularly good on cabbage or cauliflower.

¼ cup (40 g) onion, chopped

¾ cup (175 ml) white wine vinegar

2 tablespoon (30 ml) olive oil

2½ tablespoons (22.5 g) poppy seeds

1 tablespoon (13 g) sugar

1 teaspoon dry mustard

¾ cup (175 ml) olive oil

—

Yield: 12 servings

Combine first 6 ingredients in container of electric blender; blend well. Slowly add ¾ cup (175 ml) oil, continuing to blend until thick. Pour into a jar with a tight-fitting lid and chill. Shake well before serving.

NUTRITIONAL ANALYSIS

EACH WITH: 17 g water; 0 g Protein; 17 g total fat; 2 g saturated fat; 12 g monounsaturated fat; 2 g polyunsaturated fat; 2 g carb; 0 g fiber; 2 g sugar; 18 mg phosphorous; 29 mg calcium; 0 mg iron; 2 mg sodium; 30 mg potassium; 0 IU vitamin A; 0 mg ATE vitamin E; 0 mg vitamin C; 0 mg cholesterol

Pasta and Kidney Bean Salad

383 CALORIES (69% FROM FAT, 8% FROM PROTEIN, 24% FROM CARB)

This is really an easy salad to put together, especially if you're like me and tend to cook a whole pound of kidney beans while you are doing it, and then wonder what to do with the leftovers.

2 cups (270 g) rotini or other medium sized pasta

2 cups (200 g) red kidney beans, cooked

1 cup (120 g) zucchini, diced

1 cup (150 g) green bell pepper, diced

1 cup (180 g) tomato, chopped

⅓ cup (34 g) green olives, chopped

1 cup (225 g) mayonnaise

½ teaspoon chili powder

½ teaspoon coriander

½ teaspoon paprika

¼ teaspoon sage

—
Yield: 6 servings

Cook pasta until al dente. Rinse and drain. Put in large bowl and add rest of the ingredients. Mix thoroughly and serve at room temperature.

NUTRITIONAL ANALYSIS

EACH WITH: 130 g water; 8 g Protein; 30 g total fat; 5 g saturated fat; 8 g monounsaturated fat; 16 g polyunsaturated fat; 23 g carb; 8 g fiber; 2 g sugar; 129 mg phosphorous; 65 mg calcium; 3 mg iron; 423 mg sodium; 436 mg potassium; 641 IU vitamin A; 29 mg ATE vitamin E; 28 mg vitamin C; 14 mg cholesterol

TIP

You can enhance the Mediterranean feel of this salad by crumbling a little feta cheese over it.

Marinated Green Beans

173 CALORIES (68% FROM FAT, 6% FROM PROTEIN, 26% FROM CARB)

These beans make a great ingredient to liven up an otherwise ordinary salad. They also can be used as a side dish or for nibbling.

2 cups (200 g) fresh green beans

½ cup (80 g) onion, sliced

2 tablespoons (30 ml) olive oil

1 tablespoon (1.5 ml) white wine vinegar

1 teaspoon Dijon mustard

2 garlic cloves, pressed

—

Yield: 2 servings

Wash the beans; cut off the ends and break in half. Steam them for a few minutes but do not let them lose their crunchiness. Drain. Place in a salad bowl with the onions. Combine the rest of the ingredients in a jar and shake well. Pour over the beans. Serve either hot or cold.

NUTRITIONAL ANALYSIS

EACH WITH: 144 g water; 3 g Protein; 14 g total fat; 2 g saturated fat; 10 g monounsaturated fat; 2 g polyunsaturated fat; 12 g carb; 5 g fiber; 3 g sugar; 57 mg phosphorous; 52 mg calcium; 1 mg iron; 37 mg sodium; 297 mg potassium; 762 IU vitamin A; 0 mg ATE vitamin E; 21 mg vitamin C; 0 mg cholesterol

Marinated Mushrooms

118 CALORIES (74% FROM FAT, 11% FROM PROTEIN, 15% FROM CARB)

Serve these mushrooms over lettuce leaves for a tasty salad or heat them and serve with grilled beef or chicken.

1 pound (455 g) small mushrooms, cleaned

3 tablespoons (45 ml) olive oil

2 tablespoons (30 ml) lemon juice

½ teaspoon salt

½ teaspoon thyme

2 garlic cloves, chopped

½ teaspoon black pepper

2 tablespoons (8 g) fresh parsley

—
Yield: 4 servings

Slice off mushroom stems; leave the caps whole. Place in a pot with a small amount of water and cook gently for 15 minutes. Drain. Combine the remaining ingredients. Place mushrooms in the marinade and let sit for at least 2 hours in the refrigerator, stirring occasionally.

NUTRITIONAL ANALYSIS

EACH WITH: 113 g water; 4 g Protein; 11 g total fat; 1 g saturated fat; 7 g monounsaturated fat; 1 g polyunsaturated fat; 5 g carb; 1 g fiber; 2 g sugar; 100 mg phosphorous; 10 mg calcium; 1 mg iron; 302 mg sodium; 385 mg potassium; 165 IU vitamin A; 0 mg ATE vitamin E; 9 mg vitamin C; 0 mg cholesterol

Tomato, Cucumber, and Red Onion Salad with Mint

110 CALORIES (55% FROM FAT, 6% FROM PROTEIN, 39% FROM CARB)

Mint adds a refreshing note to the salad.

2 large English hothouse cucumbers

⅓ cup (80 ml) red wine vinegar

1 tablespoon (13 g) sugar

1 teaspoon salt

3 large tomatoes, seeded and coarsely chopped

⅔ cup (107 g) coarsely chopped red onion

½ cup (48 g) chopped fresh mint

3 tablespoons (45 ml) olive oil

—

Yield: 6 servings

Cut cucumbers in half lengthwise and scrape out the seeds. Cut the halves diagonally into ½-inch-wide (1 cm wide) pieces and place in a large bowl. Add vinegar, sugar, and salt and let stand at room temperature for 1 hour, tossing occasionally. Add tomatoes, red onion, mint, and oil to the cucumbers and toss to blend. Season to taste with salt and pepper.

NUTRITIONAL ANALYSIS

EACH WITH: 201 g water; 2 g protein; 7 g total fat; 1 g saturated fat; 5 g monounsaturated fat; 1 g polyunsaturated fat; 11 g carb; 2 g fiber; 7 g sugar; 53 mg phosphorus; 44 mg calcium; 1 mg iron; 402 mg sodium; 395 mg potassium; 1,034 IU vitamin A; 15 mg vitamin C; 0 mg cholesterol

Asian Chicken Pasta Salad

423 CALORIES (22% FROM FAT, 31% FROM PROTEIN, 46% FROM CARB)

This Asian flavored salad is really a full meal, and it's full of flavor.

8 ounces (225 g) orzo or other small pasta

3 tablespoons (45 ml) red wine vinegar

1½ tablespoons (30 g) chili sauce (see recipe in chapter 2)

1 tablespoon (15 ml) Reduced-Sodium Soy Sauce (see recipe in chapter 2)

1 tablespoon (15 ml) sesame oil

1 tablespoon (8 g) gingerroot, peeled and grated

2 teaspoons (10 ml) Reduced-Sodium Teriyaki Sauce (see recipe in chapter 2)

2 cups (280 g) cooked chicken breast, cubed

4 ounces (115 g) fresh spinach, sliced into strips

½ cup (25 g) bean sprouts

½ cup (75 g) red bell pepper, cut into strips

¼ cup (25 g) green onion, sliced

3 tablespoons (21 g) slivered almonds, toasted

—
Yield: 4 servings

Prepare pasta according to package directions; drain and transfer to bowl. Meanwhile, in small bowl, mix together vinegar, chili sauce, soy sauce, oil, ginger, and teriyaki sauce; whisk well. To pasta in bowl, add chicken, spinach, sprouts, bell pepper, and green onions; toss to combine. Toss dressing with pasta mixture; refrigerate 2 hours or until ready to serve. Sprinkle with almonds.

NUTRITIONAL ANALYSIS

EACH WITH: 136 g water; 33 g Protein; 10 g total fat; 2 g saturated fat; 4 g monounsaturated fat; 3 g polyunsaturated fat; 49 g carb; 4 g fiber; 4 g sugar; 335 mg phosphorous; 95 mg calcium; 4 mg iron; 115 mg sodium; 525 mg potassium; 4174 IU vitamin A; 4 mg ATE vitamin E; 27 mg vitamin C; 60 mg cholesterol

Pizza Salad

297 CALORIES (25% FROM FAT, 14% FROM PROTEIN, 61% FROM CARB)

If you have a taste for pizza but are trying to get your recommended vegetables in for the day, this salad topped pizza may be the solution you are looking for.

3 large tomatoes

½ cup (60 g) mozzarella cheese, shredded

2 tablespoons (10 g) parmesan cheese, grated

1 pizza crust, unbaked

2 cups (110 g) romaine lettuce, shredded

½ cup (75 g) red bell peppers, chopped

¼ cup (25 g) ripe olives, sliced

2 tablespoons (30 ml) Italian salad dressing

—

Yield: 6 servings

Preheat oven to 450°F (230°C, gas mark 8). Core tomatoes; slice into ¼-inch-thick (0.6 cm thick) slices and set aside. Sprinkle mozzarella and Parmesan cheeses evenly over pizza shell; top with tomato slices, slightly overlapping. Bake about 8 minutes or until cheese melts. Meanwhile, in medium bowl, combine romaine, peppers, and olives; sprinkle with Italian dressing; toss to coat. Remove pizza from oven; top with romaine mixture. Cut into wedges and serve immediately.

NUTRITIONAL ANALYSIS

EACH WITH: 108 g water; 10 g Protein; 8 g total fat; 3 g saturated fat; 3 g monounsaturated fat; 2 g polyunsaturated fat; 45 g carb; 2 g fiber; 1 g sugar; 75 mg phosphorous; 85 mg calcium; 1 mg iron; 779 mg sodium; 243 mg potassium; 1857 IU vitamin A; 19 mg ATE vitamin E; 39 mg vitamin C; 9 mg cholesterol

Chick Pea and Rice Salad

176 CALORIES (32% FROM FAT, 11% FROM PROTEIN, 57% FROM CARB)

I really like the flavor of this salad, but perhaps that's because I like the taste of cumin, which is the main spice in the dressing.

¾ cup (123 g) chick peas, cooked

1 cup (165 g) rice, cooked

½ cup (75 g) red bell pepper, diced

½ cup (75 g) green bell pepper, diced

½ cup (75 g) yellow bell pepper, diced

¼ cup (25 g) green onions, sliced

2 teaspoons (5.4 g) sesame seeds, toasted

1 teaspoon sesame oil

½ teaspoon cumin

2 tablespoons (30 ml) lemon juice

1 tablespoon (15 ml) olive oil

—

Yield: 4 servings

Toss together chick peas, rice, bell peppers, and onions in a large bowl. Whisk together all the remaining ingredients. Toss with salad.

NUTRITIONAL ANALYSIS

EACH WITH: 136 g water; 5 g Protein; 6 g total fat; 1 g saturated fat; 3 g monounsaturated fat; 2 g polyunsaturated fat; 26 g carb; 4 g fiber; 3 g sugar; 102 mg phosphorous; 49 mg calcium; 2 mg iron; 7 mg sodium; 312 mg potassium; 820 IU vitamin A; 0 mg ATE vitamin E; 129 mg vitamin C; 0 mg cholesterol

Beet and Potato Salad

103 CALORIES (36% FROM FAT, 8% FROM PROTEIN, 56% FROM CARB)

This was an experiment that turned out well. Our garden produced lots of beets this year, and I was looking for a new way to use them. Since we like them with mayonnaise, I thought of this nontraditional salad.

4 medium beets

2 large red potatoes

2 tablespoons (28 g) mayonnaise

1 tablespoon (11 g) prepared yellow mustard

—

Yield: 6 servings

Fill a large pot with water and add beets. Bring to a boil over medium-high heat and cook for about 30 minutes. Add potatoes to the water, and continue to cook until both beets and potatoes are soft, about 30 minutes more. Drain and let the vegetables cool until cool enough to handle. Cut into cubes and place them in a bowl. Stir in mayonnaise and mustard until well coated. Serve either warm or cold.

NUTRITIONAL ANALYSIS

EACH WITH: 58 g water; 2 g protein; 4 g total fat; 1 g saturated fat; 1 g monounsaturated fat; 2 g polyunsaturated fat; 15 g carb; 3 g fiber; 4 g sugar; 26 mg calcium; 2 mg iron; 48 mg sodium; 303 mg potassium; 34 IU vitamin A; 5 mg vitamin C; 3 mg cholesterol

Eggplant and Pepper Salad

136 CALORIES (77% FROM FAT, 4% FROM PROTEIN, 20% FROM CARB)

This tasty salad features roasted vegetables for a nice flavor boost. You can serve it as is over lettuce leaves. It's equally good cold or at room temperature.

1 large eggplant

2 green bell peppers

2 celery stalks

5 tablespoons (75 ml) olive oil, divided

2 garlic cloves, minced

¼ cup (60 ml) red wine vinegar

1 teaspoon oregano

½ teaspoon black pepper

¼ cup (25 g) black olives, chopped

—

Yield: 6 servings

Preheat oven to 400°F (200°C, or gas mark 6). Place whole eggplant, unpeeled, on a rack in oven. Wrap the two peppers and celery stalks individually in aluminum foil and place them on the rack as well. Bake for 30 minutes. Remove peppers and celery and let cool. Bake eggplant for another 15 minutes. It should be very tender and have collapsed. When vegetables are cool enough to handle, peel eggplant, cut into several pieces, and drain in a colander for 20 minutes. Squeeze out some of the excess moisture. Chop peppers, removing stems and seeds. Leave in large pieces. Chop celery into ½-inch (1 cm) pieces. Dice eggplant and combine with peppers and celery in a large bowl. Heat 1 tablespoon of olive oil in a skillet and sauté the garlic until golden. Add to the bowl. Add remaining ingredients and mix thoroughly. Cover and let stand for 1 hour at room temperature before serving.

NUTRITIONAL ANALYSIS

EACH WITH: 127 g water; 1 g Protein; 12 g total fat; 2 g saturated fat; 9 g monounsaturated fat; 1 g polyunsaturated fat; 7 g carb; 4 g fiber; 3 g sugar; 30 mg phosphorous; 23 mg calcium; 1 mg iron; 59 mg sodium; 272 mg potassium; 231 IU vitamin A; 0 mg ATE vitamin E; 32 mg vitamin C; 0 mg cholesterol

Double Apple Salad

160 CALORIES (52% FROM FAT, 5% FROM PROTEIN, 43% FROM CARB)

This salad has crispy apples and lots of other good things. It's hard to believe that it's actually good for you.

1 large Golden Delicious apple, diced

1 large Red Delicious apple, diced

1 teaspoon lemon juice

1 can pineapple (21 ounces or 588 g) tidbits, drained

1 cup (50 g) miniature marshmallows

⅔ cup (60 g) flaked coconut

½ cup (60 g) chopped walnuts

¼ cup (110 g) raisins

¼ cup (60 g) mayonnaise

2 tablespoons (15 g) thinly sliced celery

—
Yield: 10 servings

In a bowl, toss apples with lemon juice. Add remaining ingredients and mix well. Cover and chill for at least 1 hour.

NUTRITIONAL ANALYSIS

EACH WITH: 56 g water; 2 g protein; 10 g total fat; 2 g saturated fat; 2 g monounsaturated fat; 5 g polyunsaturated fat; 18 g carb; 1 g fiber; 13 g sugar; 48 mg phosphorus; 17 mg calcium; 1 mg iron; 39 mg sodium; 149 mg potassium; 46 IU vitamin A; 5 mg vitamin C; 2 mg cholesterol

CHAPTER 10

Side Dishes

Side dishes can be either good news or bad news from a GI standpoint. You'll want to limit the number of high-GI items like potatoes that you eat. But lots of great low-GI choices can be made. Having two vegetable dishes rather than a veggie and a starch will lower the total GI count of a meal significantly. Make that second dish a nice creamy casserole and you won't even miss the potatoes. But you don't need to give up starches completely. There also are some rice and grain dishes here that can fit into your low-GI diet, as long as you are careful with quantities.

Cauliflower Au Gratin

80 CALORIES (44% FROM FAT, 26% FROM PROTEIN, 31% FROM CARB)

This cheesy cauliflower dish is great with just about any meat. Baking allows the cheese flavor to soak even more deeply into the cauliflower.

2 cups (200 g) cauliflower, cut into pieces

1 teaspoon unsalted butter

1 teaspoon flour

1 cup (235 g) milk, cold

¼ cup (30 g) cheddar cheese, diced

½ teaspoon fresh ground pepper

—

Yield: 4 Servings

Steam cauliflower until tender. Rinse with cold water. Melt butter in saucepan. Add remaining ingredients. Cook over low heat, stirring constantly, until slightly thickened. Place cauliflower in baking dish coated with vegetable cooking spray. Cover with cheese topping. Bake at 350°F (180°C, gas mark 4) for 20 minutes.

NUTRITIONAL ANALYSIS

EACH WITH: 117 g water; 5 g Protein; 4 g total fat; 2 g saturated fat; 1 g monounsaturated fat; 0 g polyunsaturated fat; 6 g carb; 2 g fiber; 4 g sugar; 125 mg phosphorous; 148 mg calcium; 0 mg iron; 87 mg sodium; 196 mg potassium; 245 IU vitamin A; 67 mg ATE vitamin E; 28 mg vitamin C; 12 mg cholesterol

Sweet Potato Latkes

168 CALORIES (47% FROM FAT, 14% FROM PROTEIN, 39% FROM CARB)

They aren't exactly the traditional Jewish treat, but they are very tasty and sport a much lower GI index.

2 medium sweet potatoes, finely grated

3 eggs

1 teaspoon granulated sugar

4 tablespoons (24 g) almonds, finely ground

2 tablespoons (18 g) golden raisins

2 tablespoons (22 g) dates, chopped

¼ cup (28 g) pecans, chopped

—

Yield: 6 servings

In large bowl, combine sweet potatoes, eggs, sugar, and enough ground almonds to make thick batter. Mix well. Fold in raisins, dates, and pecans. In large skillet, heat ¼ inch (5 mm) oil to 375°F (190°C). Spoon a heaping tablespoon of potato mixture into oil, flattening with back of wet spoon. Brown on both sides, about 3 minutes per side. Drain on paper towels.

NUTRITIONAL ANALYSIS

EACH WITH: 63 g water; 6 g Protein; 9 g total fat; 1 g saturated fat; 5 g monounsaturated fat; 2 g polyunsaturated fat; 17 g carb; 3 g fiber; 9 g sugar; 117 mg phosphorous; 48 mg calcium; 1 mg iron; 55 mg sodium; 263 mg potassium; 8062 IU vitamin A; 39 mg ATE vitamin E; 7 mg vitamin C; 118 mg cholesterol

Bulgur and Vegetables

94 CALORIES (7% FROM FAT, 19% FROM PROTEIN, 74% FROM CARB)

In this recipe, bulgur cooked with vegetables and just enough herbs to give it a great, rich flavor. It's perfect with any kind of simple meat.

1 cup (70 g) mushrooms, fresh sliced

1 cup (120 g) zucchini, sliced quartered

1 cup (235 ml) low-sodium chicken broth

½ cup (70 g) bulgur

⅓ cup (53 g) onion, chopped

⅓ cup (37 g) carrots, chopped

¼ cup (38 g) green pepper, chopped

1 clove garlic, minced

½ teaspoon basil, dried crushed

¼ teaspoon celery seed

¼ teaspoon thyme

Dash of pepper

½ cup (90 g) tomato, chopped

—
Yield: 4 servings

In a medium saucepan, combine mushrooms, zucchini, broth, bulgur wheat, onion, green pepper, garlic, basil, celery seed, thyme, and pepper. Bring to a boil. Reduce heat and stir in chopped tomato. Let stand 5 minutes or until all the liquid is absorbed. Fluff the bulgur wheat mixture with a fork.

NUTRITIONAL ANALYSIS

EACH WITH: 152 g water; 5 g Protein; 1 g total fat; 0 g saturated fat; 0 g monounsaturated fat; 0 g polyunsaturated fat; 19 g carb; 5 g fiber; 3 g sugar; 113 mg phosphorous; 29 mg calcium; 1 mg iron; 34 mg sodium; 380 mg potassium; 2057 IU vitamin A; 0 mg ATE vitamin E; 17 mg vitamin C; 0 mg cholesterol

Country Rice

48 CALORIES (9% FROM FAT,
19% FROM PROTEIN, 72% FROM CARB)

This recipe is very similar to a rice pilaf. I'd caution against adding too many other vegetables and ending up with jambalaya instead of a side dish.

1 cup (235 ml) low-sodium chicken broth

⅔ cup (67 g) chopped green onion

¼ teaspoon black pepper

⅔ cup (130 g) uncooked rice

—

Yield: 4 servings

Bring the broth to a boil with the green onion and pepper. Add the rice, turn down to a simmer, cover, and cook for 20 minutes.

NUTRITIONAL ANALYSIS

EACH WITH: 91 g water; 2 g protein; 0 g total fat; 0 g saturated fat; 0 g monounsaturated fat; 0 g polyunsaturated fat; 9 g carb; 1 g fiber; 0 g sugar; 39 mg phosphorus; 20 mg calcium; 1 mg iron; 21 mg sodium; 114 mg potassium; 167 IU vitamin A; 3 mg vitamin C; 0 mg cholesterol

Sun-Dried Tomato Rice

85 CALORIES (55% FROM FAT,
5% FROM PROTEIN, 40% FROM CARB)

I guess I just get bored easily, but I'm always looking for a way to make things a little different. Don't get me wrong—I love plain rice. I could make a meal on a nice bowlful fresh from the steamer with nothing on it at all. But somehow that seems too plain for a meal. So we added a few Italian things to give you a different side dish. I served it with a grilled piece of fish that had been marinated in Italian dressing.

¼ cup (40 g) chopped onion

1 cup (195 g) uncooked rice

2 tablespoons (30 ml) olive oil

¼ teaspoon garlic powder

¼ cup (14 g) chopped sun-dried tomatoes

2¼ cups (535 ml) water

—

Yield: 6 servings

Sauté onion and rice in oil about 2 minutes or until rice begins to brown. Add remaining ingredients, cover, reduce heat, and simmer 20 minutes or until rice is tender.

NUTRITIONAL ANALYSIS

EACH WITH: 116 g water; 1 g protein; 5 g total fat; 1 g saturated fat; 4 g monounsaturated fat; 1 g polyunsaturated fat; 9 g carb; 1 g fiber; 0 g sugar; 23 mg phosphorus; 11 mg calcium; 1 mg iron; 16 mg sodium; 98 mg potassium; 59 IU vitamin A; 5 mg vitamin C; 0 mg cholesterol

Spicy Rice

237 CALORIES (63% FROM FAT, 14% FROM PROTEIN, 23% FROM CARB)

This dish is a family favorite. It's a quick and flavorful use for leftover rice.

1 cup (220 g) cooked brown rice

2 tablespoons (30 ml) olive oil

½ cup (80 g) chopped onion

¼ pound (115 g) shredded cheddar cheese

1 jalapeño pepper, chopped

—

Yield: 4 servings

Brown rice in oil. Add remaining ingredients. Cover and simmer until heated through and cheese is melted.

NUTRITIONAL ANALYSIS

EACH WITH: 67 g water; 9 g protein; 17 g total fat; 7 g saturated fat; 8 g monounsaturated fat; 1 g polyunsaturated fat; 14 g carb; 1 g fiber; 1 g sugar; 192 mg phosphorus; 214 mg calcium; 1 mg iron; 179 mg sodium; 86 mg potassium; 312 IU vitamin A; 3 mg vitamin C; 30 mg cholesterol

Easy Curried Vegetables

43 CALORIES (9% FROM FAT, 16% FROM PROTEIN, 75% FROM CARB)

Many Indian curry recipes involve frying the spices first to develop a richer flavor. This recipe uses a simpler preparation method but still gives you flavorful vegetables to go with whatever meat you are serving.

2 cups (480 g) no-salt-added canned tomatoes

2 cups (226 g) sliced zucchini

½ cup (80 g) coarsely chopped onion

1 tablespoon (6 g) curry powder

—
Yield: 4 servings

Combine ingredients in a saucepan. Cook over medium heat until onion and zucchini are tender.

NUTRITIONAL ANALYSIS

EACH WITH: 190 g water; 2 g protein; 1 g total fat; 0 g saturated fat; 0 g monounsaturated fat; 0 g polyunsaturated fat; 10 g carb; 3 g fiber; 5 g sugar; 58 mg phosphorus; 59 mg calcium; 2 mg iron; 23 mg sodium; 442 mg potassium; 280 IU vitamin A; 23 mg vitamin C; 0 mg cholesterol

Roasted Vegetables

149 CALORIES (3% FROM FAT, 12% FROM PROTEIN, 86% FROM CARB)

Here's a simple but tasty way to cook vegetables.

3 potatoes, cubed

1 cup (130 g) carrot,
sliced 1 inch (2½ cm) long

½ cup (75 g) green bell pepper,
cut in chunks

½ cup (75 g) red bell pepper,
cut in chunks

4 ounces (115 g) mushrooms

½ teaspoon onion powder

¼ teaspoon garlic powder

½ teaspoon thyme

—
Yield: 6 servings

Place vegetables in a single layer in a roasting pan. Coat with nonstick olive oil spray. Sprinkle with spices. Roast at 350°F (180°C, gas mark 4) until done, about 30 minutes, turning once.

NUTRITIONAL ANALYSIS

EACH WITH: 209 g water; 5 g protein; 0 g total fat; 0 g saturated fat; 0 g monounsaturated fat; 0 g polyunsaturated fat; 34 g carb; 4 g fiber; 4 g sugar; 143 mg phosphorus; 31 mg calcium; 2 mg iron; 28 mg sodium; 1,020 mg potassium; 4,037 IU vitamin A; 43 mg vitamin C; 0 mg cholesterol

Corn and Zucchini Bake

154 CALORIES (29% FROM FAT, 31% FROM PROTEIN, 40% FROM CARB)

Here's something a little different in a vegetable side dish, with corn and zucchini contributing to a cheese-flavored custard.

3 cups (339 g) sliced zucchini

¼ cup (40 g) chopped onion

1 tablespoon (15 ml) olive oil

10 ounces (280 g) frozen corn, cooked

1 cup (115 g) shredded low-fat Swiss cheese

2 eggs

¼ cup (30 g) bread crumbs

2 tablespoons (10 g) grated Parmesan cheese

—

Yield: 6 servings

Cook zucchini in boiling water until soft. Drain and mash with fork. Sauté onion in oil until soft. Combine zucchini, onion, corn, cheese, and eggs. Turn into a 1-quart (1 L) casserole coated with nonstick vegetable oil spray. Combine bread crumbs and Parmesan; sprinkle over top. Place on a baking sheet and bake uncovered at 350°F (180°C, gas mark 4) until a knife inserted near the center comes out clean, about 40 minutes.

NUTRITIONAL ANALYSIS

EACH WITH: 132 g water; 12 g protein; 5 g total fat; 2 g saturated fat; 2 g monounsaturated fat; 1 g polyunsaturated fat; 16 g carb; 2 g fiber; 4 g sugar; 233 mg phosphorus; 267 mg calcium; 1 mg iron; 168 mg sodium; 347 mg potassium; 243 IU vitamin A; 12 mg vitamin C; 10 mg cholesterol

Mashed Turnips

32 CALORIES (40% FROM FAT, 8% FROM PROTEIN, 52% FROM CARB)

They probably aren't something you typically think about as a side dish, but mashed turnips make a nice alternative to potatoes, with a significantly lower GI count.

1½ pounds (680 g) small turnips, peeled and quartered

Black pepper, to taste

½ teaspoon garlic, roasted and peeled

1 tablespoon (14 g) unsalted butter

Skim milk (optional)

—

Yield: 8 servings

Steam turnips over boiling water until fork tender, about 15 minutes. Drain turnips and place in a food processor or blender along with garlic and butter. Process until smooth, adding skim milk as needed.

NUTRITIONAL ANALYSIS

EACH WITH: 80 g water; 1 g Protein; 2 g total fat; 1 g saturated fat; 0 g monounsaturated fat; 0 g polyunsaturated fat; 4 g carb; 2 g fiber; 3 g sugar; 23 mg phosphorous; 29 mg calcium; 0 mg iron; 14 mg sodium; 152 mg potassium; 44 IU vitamin A; 12 mg ATE vitamin E; 10 mg vitamin C; 4 mg cholesterol

CHAPTER 11

Low-GI Breads and Baked Goods

Breads and baked goods are by their very nature higher in GI than many foods. Most consist primarily of flour and sugar. We've reduced the GI count of the ones in this chapter by relying mostly on whole grain flours and by replacing the sugar with a sweetener like Splenda. You'll still need to be aware of how much you eat, but you don't need to give these kinds of foods up completely.

Oatmeal Bread

167 CALORIES (13% FROM FAT, 15% FROM PROTEIN, 72% FROM CARB)

This bread has a wonderful, slightly sweet flavor. It's great toasted for breakfast or for sandwiches.

1 cup (80 g) quick-cooking oats

⅔ cup (160 ml) skim milk

⅓ cup (80 ml) water

1 tablespoon (14 g) unsalted butter

½ cup (60 g) whole wheat flour

2 cups (275 g) bread flour

3 tablespoons (3 g) brown sugar substitute, such as Splenda

1 teaspoon yeast

—
Yield: 12 servings

Spread the oats in a baking pan and toast in an oven heated to 350°F (180°C, gas mark 4) until lightly browned, about 15 minutes, stirring occasionally. Place ingredients in bread machine in order specified by manufacturer. Process on whole grain cycle.

NUTRITIONAL ANALYSIS

EACH WITH: 24 g water; 6 g protein; 2 g total fat; 1 g saturated fat; 1 g monounsaturated fat; 1 g polyunsaturated fat; 30 g carb; 3 g fiber; 1 g sugar; 127 mg phosphorus; 32 mg calcium; 2 mg iron; 10 mg sodium; 131 mg potassium; 58 IU vitamin A; 0 mg vitamin C; 3 mg cholesterol

Italian Peasant Bread

146 CALORIES (18% FROM FAT, 13% FROM PROTEIN, 69% FROM CARB)

This is a recipe we've been using for a while and our favorite for Italian bread. I use the bread machine to make my dough and then bake it in the oven to get that traditional look.

2 cups (275 g) bread flour

1 cup (120 g) whole wheat flour

2 tablespoons (30 ml) olive oil

2 teaspoons sugar substitute, such as Splenda

2 teaspoons active dry yeast

1 cup (235 ml) warm water

2 tablespoons (18 g) cornmeal, for baking sheet

1 egg white, slightly beaten

—

Yield: 12 servings

Add flour, oil, salt, sugar, yeast, and water to your bread machine according to its instructions. Set on dough setting. Remove when signal beeps and cycle is done. Preheat oven to 375°F (190°C, gas mark 5). Sprinkle cornmeal onto a baking sheet. Punch dough down and form into a long or oval loaf. Cover and let rise for 25 more minutes. It should be doubled again by this time. Uncover and slash the top with a sharp knife or razor. Brush all over with the beaten egg white. Bake 25 to 35 minutes until hollow sounding when tapped on bottom.

NUTRITIONAL ANALYSIS

EACH WITH: 26 g water; 5 g protein; 3 g total fat; 0 g saturated fat; 2 g monounsaturated fat; 0 g polyunsaturated fat; 26 g carb; 2 g fiber; 0 g sugar; 68 mg phosphorus; 8 mg calcium; 2 mg iron; 7 mg sodium; 84 mg potassium; 5 IU vitamin A; 0 mg vitamin C; 0 mg cholesterol

Whole Wheat Pizza Dough

119 CALORIES (16% FROM FAT, 12% FROM PROTEIN, 71% FROM CARB)

We used this dough to make a pizza full of fresh veggies from the garden, but you could use it with any toppings you desire.

2 teaspoons (8 g) active dry yeast

2 cups (275) bread flour

1½ cups (180 g) whole wheat flour

1 tablespoon (13 g) sugar substitute, such as Splenda

2 tablespoons (30 ml) olive oil

1½ cups (355 ml) water

—
Yield: 16 servings

Place ingredients in bread machine in order specified by manufacturer and process on dough cycle. Turn out the dough onto a floured board. At this point you may form the pizzas or refrigerate the dough for several hours, well wrapped in plastic so it won't dry out. It makes enough dough for two 12-inch (30 cm) pizzas or two 10-inch (25 cm) thick-crust pizzas. Bake at 400°F (200°C, gas mark 6) until lightly browned around the edges. Top as desired and return to oven until cheese is melted and crust browned, about 15 minutes total.

NUTRITIONAL ANALYSIS

EACH WITH: 26 g water; 4 g protein; 2 g total fat; 0 g saturated fat; 1 g monounsaturated fat; 0 g polyunsaturated fat; 22 g carb; 2 g fiber; 1 g sugar; 62 mg phosphorus; 7 mg calcium; 1 mg iron; 2 mg sodium; 73 mg potassium; 1 IU vitamin A; 0 mg vitamin C; 0 mg cholesterol

Chili Cheese Corn Bread

88 CALORIES (21% FROM FAT, 17% FROM PROTEIN, 63% FROM CARB)

Unlike the corn muffin recipe, which goes with any kind of meal, this corn bread begs to be eaten with Mexican food, with its chili and cheese flavors.

1 cup (140 g) yellow cornmeal

2 teaspoons (9.2 g) baking powder

½ teaspoon baking soda

¼ cup (150 g) whole wheat flour

1¼ cups (285 ml) buttermilk

1 egg, lightly beaten

1 egg white, lightly beaten

¼ cup (30 g) cheddar, shredded

2 tablespoons (15 g) mild green chilies

—

Yield: 12 servings

Preheat oven to 450°F (230°C, or gas mark 8). Coat an 8 × 8-inch (20 × 20 cm) baking pan with nonstick cooking spray and dust with cornmeal. Sift into a large bowl the cornmeal, baking powder, baking soda, and flour. In another bowl, combine buttermilk, eggs, cheese, and chilies, then stir into the dry ingredients. Pour batter into the prepared baking pan and place in upper third of oven. Bake 10 minutes or until dough is firm in center.

NUTRITIONAL ANALYSIS

EACH WITH: 32 g water; 4 g Protein; 2 g total fat; 1 g saturated fat; 1 g monounsaturated fat; 0 g polyunsaturated fat; 14 g carb; 1 g fiber; 2 g sugar; 85 mg phosphorous; 99 mg calcium; 1 mg iron; 144 mg sodium; 83 mg potassium; 93 IU vitamin A; 16 mg ATE vitamin E; 1 mg vitamin C; 21 mg cholesterol

Pumpkin Pancakes

194 CALORIES (29% FROM FAT, 13% FROM PROTEIN, 59% FROM CARB)

Pumpkin, rather than the usual amount of sugar, sweetens these pancakes. I like them just as is or maybe with a little cottage cheese.

1 egg

1 cup (235 ml) milk

½ cup (123 g) pumpkin, cooked or canned

¾ cup (94 g) flour

¾ cup (90 g) whole wheat flour

2 teaspoons (9.2 g) baking powder

1 tablespoon sugar substitute, such as Splenda

¼ teaspoon cinnamon

⅛ teaspoon nutmeg

⅛ teaspoon ginger

2 tablespoons (10 ml) canola oil

—

Yield: 6 servings

Combine all the ingredients in a mixing bowl and stir just until blended. Pour the batter onto a hot griddle that has been lightly oiled. Flip the pancakes over when bubbles break around the edges.

NUTRITIONAL ANALYSIS

EACH WITH: 64 g water; 6 g Protein; 6 g total fat; 1 g saturated fat; 3 g monounsaturated fat; 2 g polyunsaturated fat; 29 g carb; 3 g fiber; 5 g sugar; 167 mg phosphorous; 160 mg calcium; 2 mg iron; 197 mg sodium; 196 mg potassium; 3318 IU vitamin A; 40 mg ATE vitamin E; 1 mg vitamin C; 36 mg cholesterol

Carrot Cake Muffins

125 CALORIES (32% FROM FAT, 11% FROM PROTEIN, 56% FROM CARB)

Carrot cake is one of my favorite desserts, but I don't have it very often because it tends to be high in carbohydrates and other not so healthy stuff. These muffins are a bit better, giving a healthy dose of fruits and vegetables and a reasonable low GI.

1½ cups (180 g) whole wheat flour

1 teaspoon baking soda

1 tablespoon (13.8 g) baking powder

1 teaspoon ground cinnamon

¼ teaspoon ground nutmeg

¼ teaspoon ground ginger

1 egg

2 tablespoons (30 ml) vegetable oil

¼ cup (36 g) raisins

¼ cup (30 g) walnuts, chopped

⅓ cup (80 ml) skim milk

8 ounces (225 g) crushed pineapple

1½ cups (165 g) carrots, grated

—
Yield: 12 servings

Combine the dry ingredients in a bowl. Add the remaining ingredients and stir to blend. Spoon into oiled muffin tins or paper muffin cups. Bake at 350°F (180°C, or gas mark 4) for 20 to 25 minutes.

NUTRITIONAL ANALYSIS

EACH WITH: 41 g water; 4 g Protein; 5 g total fat; 1 g saturated fat; 1 g monounsaturated fat; 2 g polyunsaturated fat; 19 g carb; 3 g fiber; 5 g sugar; 117 mg phosphorous; 98 mg calcium; 1 mg iron; 146 mg sodium; 191 mg potassium; 2742 IU vitamin A; 12 mg ATE vitamin E; 3 mg vitamin C; 18 mg cholesterol

Blueberry Buttermilk Muffins

97 CALORIES (41% FROM FAT, 11% FROM PROTEIN, 48% FROM CARB)

Blueberries and strawberries have both been on sale around here lately, so I decided it had been too long since I'd had fresh blueberry muffins. This one makes a big batch, so the family doesn't need to argue over the last one.

2½ cups (300 g) whole wheat pastry flour

1½ teaspoons baking powder

½ teaspoon baking soda

¾ cup (18 g) sugar substitute, such as Splenda

2 eggs

1 cup (235 ml) buttermilk

4 ounces (112 g) unsalted butter

1½ cups (120 g) blueberries

—

Yield: 24 muffins

Sift dry ingredients together in a large bowl. In another bowl, whisk eggs, buttermilk, and butter that has been melted and browned slightly. Make a well in dry ingredients and pour in liquid ingredients, mixing quickly. Fold in blueberries. Spoon batter into greased muffin cups and bake at 400°F (200°C, gas mark 6) for 20 to 30 minutes until golden brown.

NUTRITIONAL ANALYSIS

EACH WITH: 23 g water; 3 g protein; 5 g total fat; 3 g saturated fat; 1 g monounsaturated fat; 0 g polyunsaturated fat; 12 g carb; 2 g fiber; 3 g sugar; 70 mg phosphorus; 37 mg calcium; 1 mg iron; 49 mg sodium; 81 mg potassium; 150 IU vitamin A; 1 mg vitamin C; 30 mg cholesterol

Pizza Snack Muffins

138 CALORIES (35% FROM FAT, 17% FROM PROTEIN, 47% FROM CARB)

These are good as a snack or for those who have always wanted pizza for breakfast.

2 cups (240 g) whole wheat pastry flour

2 teaspoons baking powder

1 teaspoon basil

1 teaspoon oregano

¾ cup (175 ml) skim milk

1 egg

2 tablespoons (30 ml) olive oil

½ cup (90 g) chopped tomatoes

½ cup (75 g) finely chopped pepperoni

2¼ ounces (65 g) black olives, sliced ripe

¾ cup (90 g) shredded mozzarella cheese

—
Yield: 12 servings

In a bowl, mix flour, baking powder, basil, and oregano. Add milk, egg, and oil; stir to moisten. Add tomatoes, pepperoni, olives, and half of the cheese; mix well. Divide batter equally among 10 oiled muffin cups (2 to 2½ inches or 5 to 6 cm); top with remaining cheese. Bake in oven heated to 350°F (180°C, gas mark 4) until muffins are well browned, 30 to 35 minutes. Let stand about 5 minutes and then remove from pan. Serve warm or cool.

NUTRITIONAL ANALYSIS

EACH WITH: 37 g water; 6 g protein; 6 g total fat; 2 g saturated fat; 3 g monounsaturated fat; 1 g polyunsaturated fat; 17 g carb; 3 g fiber; 1 g sugar; 158 mg phosphorus; 147 mg calcium; 1 mg iron; 189 mg sodium; 149 mg potassium; 119 IU vitamin A; 1 mg vitamin C; 25 mg cholesterol

Cranberry Bread

149 CALORIES (35% FROM FAT, 10% FROM PROTEIN, 55% FROM CARB)

This makes a nice holiday breakfast loaf, but we like it so much that we don't wait for a holiday.

1 cup (110 g) cranberries, chopped

½ cup (55 g) pecans, chopped

1 tablespoon (6 g) grated orange peel

2 cups (240 g) whole wheat pastry flour

1 cup (25 g) sugar substitute, such as Splenda

1½ teaspoons baking powder

½ teaspoon baking soda

2 tablespoons (28 g) unsalted butter

¾ cup (175 ml) orange juice

1 egg, well beaten

—

Yield: 12 servings

Preheat oven to 350°F (180°C, or gas mark 4). Generously grease and lightly flour a 9 × 5-inch (23 × 13 cm) loaf pan. Prepare cranberries, nuts, and orange peel. Set aside. In a bowl, mix together flour, sugar, baking powder, and soda. Cut in butter. Stir in orange juice, egg, and orange peel mixing just to moisten. Fold in cranberries and nuts. Spoon into prepared pan. Bake 60 minutes or until wooden pick inserted into center comes out clean. Cool on a rack 15 minutes before removing from pan.

NUTRITIONAL ANALYSIS

EACH WITH: 28 g water; 4 g Protein; 6 g total fat; 2 g saturated fat; 3 g monounsaturated fat; 1 g polyunsaturated fat; 22 g carb; 3 g fiber; 4 g sugar; 106 mg phosphorous; 50 mg calcium; 1 mg iron; 70 mg sodium; 145 mg potassium; 111 IU vitamin A; 23 mg ATE vitamin E; 7 mg vitamin C; 23 mg cholesterol

TIP

You can buy fresh cranberries when they are in season and freeze them right in the bag they came in so you have them for recipes like this one.

CHAPTER 12

Sweets and Drinks

It's easy to find high-GI desserts. But you can limit the GI content by replacing white flour with whole wheat pastry flour and by limited the quantity you eat. Along with the cookies and cakes, we also have some good fruit desserts and a couple of tasty low-GI drinks.

Peanut Butter Cookies

62 CALORIES (67% FROM FAT, 9% FROM PROTEIN, 24% FROM CARB)

The use of sugar substitutes makes these cookies good for anyone who is watching their carbohydrates and trying to eat a lower GI diet. And the taste is every bit as good as the regular peanut butter cookies they are patterned after.

⅓ cup (42 g) flour

¼ teaspoon baking soda

¼ teaspoon baking powder

¼ cup (55 g) unsalted butter

4 tablespoons (64 g) peanut butter

1 tablespoon (1 g) brown sugar substitute, such as Splenda

½ cup (12 g) sugar substitute, such as Splenda

1 egg, well beaten

—
Yield: 18 servings

Preheat oven to 375°F (190°C, or gas mark 5). Grease cookie sheet lightly. Sift together flour, baking soda, and baking powder. Work butter and peanut butter with spoon until creamy; gradually add brown sugar replacement and continue working until light. Add granulated sugar replacement and egg; beat well. Mix in dry ingredients thoroughly. Drop by teaspoonfuls onto cookie sheet; flatten with tines of fork in a crisscross pattern. Bake until done, 8 to 10 minutes.

NUTRITIONAL ANALYSIS

EACH WITH: 3 g water; 1 g Protein; 5 g total fat; 2 g saturated fat; 2 g monounsaturated fat; 1 g polyunsaturated fat; 4 g carb; 0 g fiber; 2 g sugar; 21 mg phosphorous; 8 mg calcium; 0 mg iron; 13 mg sodium; 34 mg potassium; 97 IU vitamin A; 26 mg ATE vitamin E; 0 mg vitamin C; 18 mg cholesterol

Fudge Brownies

155 CALORIES (66% FROM FAT, 7% FROM PROTEIN, 27% FROM CARB)

Yes, you can have brownies. This quick brownie recipe gets a fiber and nutrition boost from the whole wheat flour.

1 cup (225 g) unsalted butter

½ cup (40 g) cocoa powder

2 cups (50 g) sugar substitute, such as Splenda

4 eggs

2 teaspoons (10 ml) vanilla

1 cup (120 g) whole wheat pastry flour

—
Yield: 18 servings

Heat oven to 350°F (180°C, gas mark 4). In microwave, melt butter and cocoa together, stirring once or twice. When melted, add sugar substitute, eggs, and vanilla. Stir to mix well and then add flour. Pour into greased 13 × 9-inch (33 × 23 cm) pan. Bake 25 minutes.

NUTRITIONAL ANALYSIS

EACH WITH: 13 g water; 3 g protein; 12 g total fat; 7 g saturated fat; 3 g monounsaturated fat; 1 g polyunsaturated fat; 11 g carb; 2 g fiber; 4 g sugar; 67 mg phosphorus; 15 mg calcium; 1 mg iron; 20 mg sodium; 84 mg potassium; 376 IU vitamin A; 0 mg vitamin C; 80 mg cholesterol

Apple Cake

246 CALORIES (58% FROM FAT, 9% FROM PROTEIN, 34% FROM CARB)

Everyone wants something sweet every once in a while. But that doesn't mean that it still can't still be good for you. Whole wheat flour and apples bump up the nutrition and fiber levels of this cake, but the taste just says "good."

2¼ cups (250 g) whole wheat pastry flour

1 cup (25 g) sugar substitute, such as Splenda

¾ cup (12 g) brown sugar substitute, such as Splenda

1 tablespoon (7 g) cinnamon

2 teaspoons baking powder

½ teaspoon baking soda

¾ cup (175 ml) canola oil

1 teaspoon vanilla

3 eggs

2 cups (250 g) finely chopped apple

1 cup (120 g) chopped walnuts

¼ cup (25 g) powdered sugar, sifted

—
Yield: 16 servings

Generously grease and flour a 10-inch (25 cm) fluted tube pan; set aside. In a large mixing bowl, combine the flour, sugar substitutes, cinnamon, baking powder, and baking soda. Add oil, vanilla, and the eggs; beat until well mixed. Stir in the chopped apple and walnuts. Spoon batter evenly into prepared pan. Bake in an oven heated to 350°F (180°C, gas mark 4) for 45 to 50 minutes or until cake tests done. Cool in pan 12 minutes; invert cake onto a wire rack. Cool thoroughly. Sprinkle with powdered sugar.

NUTRITIONAL ANALYSIS

EACH WITH: 23 g water; 6 g protein; 17 g total fat; 1 g saturated fat; 8 g monounsaturated fat; 6 g polyunsaturated fat; 22 g carb; 3 g fiber; 8 g sugar; 133 mg phosphorus; 56 mg calcium; 1 mg iron; 77 mg sodium; 139 mg potassium; 62 IU vitamin A; 1 mg vitamin C; 44 mg cholesterol

Lite Lemon Cheesecake

141 CALORIES (57% FROM FAT, 21% FROM PROTEIN, 22% FROM CARB)

Do you think that you can't have cheesecake on your low GI diet? Think again. This cheese-cake is full of flavor but not full of carbs or fat, so it works for just about anyone.

⅓ cup (40 g) graham cracker crumbs

1 small box sugar-free lemon gelatin

⅔ cup (160 ml) water, boiling

1 cup (225 g) fat-free cottage cheese

8 ounces (225 g) fat-free cream cheese

2 cups (150 g) whipped topping, like Cool Whip

—
Yield: 8 servings

Spray 8- or 9-inch (20 × 23 cm) springform pan or 9-inch (23 cm) pie plate lightly with nonstick cooking spray. Sprinkle with graham cracker crumbs. Completely dissolve gelatin in boiling water; pour into blender container. Add cottage cheese and cream cheese; cover. Blend at medium speed, scraping down sides occasionally, about 2 minutes or until mixture is completely smooth. Pour into large bowl. Gently stir in whipped topping. Pour into prepared pan; smooth top. Chill until set, about 4 hours.

NUTRITIONAL ANALYSIS

EACH WITH: 70 g water; 7 g Protein; 9 g total fat; 5 g saturated fat; 3 g monounsaturated fat; 0 g polyunsaturated fat; 8 g carb; 0 g fiber; 3 g sugar; 107 mg phosphorous; 66 mg calcium; 1 mg iron; 247 mg sodium; 99 mg potassium; 307 IU vitamin A; 82 mg ATE vitamin E; 0 mg vitamin C; 28 mg cholesterol

Baked Apples

106 CALORIES (2% FROM FAT, 2% FROM PROTEIN, 96% FROM CARB)

This simple baked apple recipe contains no added sugar, letting the flavor of the apples come through.

4 apples

¼ cup (36 g) raisins

½ cup (120 ml) apple juice, unsweetened

—

Yield: 4 servings

Preheat oven to 375°F (190°C, or gas mark 5). Wash and core apples. Pare a strip from top of each apple. Put tablespoon (9 g) of raisins in each apple. Pour apple juice over apples. Bake 40 minutes or until done. Baste apples with juice during cooking. Serve warm or chilled.

NUTRITIONAL ANALYSIS

EACH WITH: 139 g water;1 g Protein; 0 g total fat; 0 g saturated fat; 0 g monounsaturated fat; 0 g polyunsaturated fat; 28 g carb; 2 g fiber; 22 g sugar; 27 mg phosphorous; 13 mg calcium; 0 mg iron; 3 mg sodium; 230 mg potassium; 49 IU vitamin A; 0 mg ATE vitamin E; 6 mg vitamin C; 0 mg cholesterol

Frozen Cherry Dessert

46 CALORIES (42% FROM FAT, 13% FROM PROTEIN, 44% FROM CARB)

This frozen dessert makes a great low GI alternative to ice cream.

8 ounces (225 g) sweet cherries, undrained, pitted

1 small box sugar-free gelatin, cherry flavor

1 cup (235 g) water, boiling

8 ounces plain fat-free yogurt

2 cups (150 g) whipped topping, like Cool Whip

—

Yield: 12 servings

Line bottom and sides of 9 × 5-inch (23 × 13 cm) loaf pan with plastic wrap; set aside. Drain cherries, reserving syrup. If necessary, add enough cold water to reserved syrup to measure ½ cup (120 ml). Cut cherries into quarters. Completely dissolve gelatin in boiling water. Add measured syrup. Stir in yogurt until well blended. Chill until mixture is thickened but not set, about 45 minutes to 1 hour, stirring occasionally. Gently stir in cherries and whipped topping. Pour into prepared pan; cover. Freeze until firm, about 6 hours or overnight. Remove pan from freezer about 15 minutes before serving. Let stand at room temperature to soften slightly. Remove plastic wrap. Cut into slices. Cover and store leftovers in freezer.

NUTRITIONAL ANALYSIS

EACH WITH: 58 g water; 2 g Protein; 2 g total fat; 1 g saturated fat; 1 g monounsaturated fat; 0 g polyunsaturated fat; 5 g carb; 0 g fiber; 4 g sugar; 48 mg phosphorous; 50 mg calcium; 0 mg iron; 33 mg sodium; 88 mg potassium; 100 IU vitamin A; 19 mg ATE vitamin E; 1 mg vitamin C; 8 mg cholesterol

Lime Fizz

41 CALORIES (1% FROM FAT,
1% FROM PROTEIN, 98% FROM CARB)

If you are looking for something cool and refreshing to drink, give this a try. You can also use lemon juice to make a lemon fizz. Adjust the amount of juice and sweetener to your own taste.

2 tablespoons (30 ml) lime juice
2 teaspoons sugar substitute, such as Splenda
¼ cup (60 ml) water
1 cup (235 ml) seltzer water

—

Yield: 1 serving

Combine juice, artificial sweetener, and water in a tall glass. Stir until dissolved. Add ice. Fill glass with seltzer.

NUTRITIONAL ANALYSIS

EACH WITH: 324 g water; 0 g protein; 0 g total fat; 0 g saturated fat; 0 g monounsaturated fat; 0 g polyunsaturated fat; 11 g carb; 0 g fiber; 9 g sugar; 37 mg calcium; 0 mg iron; 4 mg sodium; 34 mg potassium; 15 IU vitamin A; 9 mg vitamin C; 0 mg cholesterol

Lemonade

24 CALORIES (0% FROM FAT,
1% FROM PROTEIN, 99% FROM CARB)

When the weather is hot, a tall cold glass of lemonade sure tastes good. Fresh-squeezed lemon juice is best, but you can still get good lemonade using bottled juice.

½ cup (100 g) sugar substitute, such as Splenda
1½ cups (355 ml) lemon juice
5 quarts (5 L) water

—

Yield: 20 servings

Heat sugar and lemon juice just until sugar dissolves. Add to water. Stir and serve over ice.

NUTRITIONAL ANALYSIS

EACH WITH: 253 g water; 0 g protein; 0 g total fat; 0 g saturated fat; 0 g monounsaturated fat; 0 g polyunsaturated fat; 7 g carb; 0 g fiber; 5 g sugar; 1 mg phosphorus; 8 mg calcium; 0 mg iron; 7 mg sodium; 25 mg potassium; 3 IU vitamin A; 8 mg vitamin C; 0 mg cholesterol

Fruit Slush

274 G WATER; 274 CALORIES (1% FROM FAT, 3% FROM PROTEIN, 96% FROM CARB)

This is sort of like sherbet but without as much preparation effort. This works either as a dessert or just a cooling snack on a hot day.

6 ounces (170 g) lemonade concentrate undiluted

6 ounces (170 g) orange juice concentrate undiluted

½ cup (12 g) sugar substitute, such as Splenda

16 ounces (475 g) lemon-lime carbonated beverage

15 ounces (425 g) crushed pineapple, drained

14 ounces (400 g) fruit cocktail

2 cups banana, sliced

—
Yield: 6 servings

Mix by hand. Freeze. Let thaw 10 minutes before serving. Stir to make slush.

NUTRITIONAL ANALYSIS

EACH WITH: 2 g Protein; 0 g total fat; 0 g saturated fat; 0 g mono-unsaturated fat; 0 g polyunsaturated fat; 70 g carb; 3 g fiber; 60 g sugar; 49 mg phosphorous; 32 mg calcium; 1 mg iron; 14 mg sodium; 617 mg potassium; 386 IU vitamin A; 0 mg ATE vitamin E; 58 mg vitamin C; 0 mg cholesterol

Cappuccino Mousse

117 CALORIES (36% FROM FAT, 10% FROM PROTEIN, 54% FROM CARB)

This is great for those times when you want a fancy dessert that no one knows has a low-GI rating.

3 cups (705 ml) 1 percent milk

1 sugar-free chocolate pudding mix

6 teaspoons (11 g) decaffeinated instant coffee

½ teaspoon cinnamon

2 cups (150 g) fat-free whipped topping

—

Yield: 10 servings

Pour milk into 5-quart (5 L) mixer bowl. Add pudding mix, instant coffee, and cinnamon. Blend by hand with a wire whip, scraping the sides of bowl to moisten completely. Whip at medium speed with electric mixer for 3 minutes or until pudding is smooth and creamy. Fold in whipped topping. Immediately portion ½ cup into stemmed glasses or coffee mugs. Chill at least 1 hour. Keep refrigerated.

NUTRITIONAL ANALYSIS

EACH WITH: 74 g water; 3 g protein; 5 g total fat; 4 g saturated fat; 1 g monounsaturated fat; 0 g polyunsaturated fat; 16 g carb; 0 g fiber; 12 g sugar; 165 mg phosphorus; 91 mg calcium; 0 mg iron; 178 mg sodium; 156 mg potassium; 165 IU vitamin A; 0 mg vitamin C; 4 mg cholesterol

About the Author

Dick Logue is the author of several cookbooks. After being diagnosed with congestive heart failure more than ten years ago, Dick threw himself into the process of creating healthy versions of his favorite recipes. A cook since the age of twelve, he grows his own vegetables, bakes his own bread, and cans a variety of foods.

He is the author of *500 Low-Sodium Recipes*, *500 Low-Cholesterol Recipes*, *500 High-Fiber Recipes*, 500 Low-Glycemic-Index Recipes, *500 Heart-Healthy Slow Cooker Recipes*, *500 400-Calorie Recipes*, and *500 15-Minute Low-Sodium Recipes*. He lives in La Plata, Maryland.

Index